'BEING ALIVE WELL'
Health and the Politics of Cree Well-Being

'Being Alive Well': Health and the Politics of Cree Well-Being is a critical anthropological analysis of health theory with specific reference to the James Bay Cree of northern Quebec. In it the author argues that definitions of health are not simply reflections of physiological soundness but convey broader cultural and political realities. The book begins with a treatise on the study of health in the social sciences and a call for a broader understanding of the cultural parameters of any definition of health. Following a chapter that outlines the history of the Whapmagoostui (Great Whale River) region and the people, Adelson presents the underlying symbolic foundations of a Cree approach to health, or *miyupimaatisiiun* ('being alive well'). The core of this book is an ethnographic study of the Whapmagoostui Cree and their particular concept of health. That concept is mediated by history, cultural practices, and the contemporary world of the Cree, including their fundamental concerns about their land and culture. In the contemporary context, health – 'being alive well' – for the Cree of Great Whale is a fusion of social, political, and personal well-being, linking individual bodies to a larger socio-political reality.

(Anthropological Horizons)

NAOMI ADELSON is Associate Professor of Anthropology at York University. She has been working with the Whapmagoostui Cree of northern Quebec since 1988 and continues to conduct research with the Cree on issues relating to social stress, community gatherings, and contemporary and historical shifts in religious and healing beliefs and practices.

'Being Alive Well'

Health and the Politics of Cree Well-Being

NAOMI ADELSON

UNIVERSITY OF TORONTO PRESS
Toronto Buffalo London

© University of Toronto Press Incorporated 2000
Toronto Buffalo London
Printed in Canada

Reprinted 2002, 2004

ISBN 0-8020-4777-7 (cloth)
ISBN 0-8020-8326-9 (paper)

∞

Printed on acid-free paper

Canadian Cataloguing in Publication Data

Adelson, Naomi, 1958–
    'Being alive well': health and the politics of Cree well-being

    Includes bibliographical references and index.
    ISBN 0-8020-4777-7 (bound)   ISBN 0-8020-8326-9 (pbk.)

    1. Cree Indians – Medicine – Quebec (Province) – Whapmagoostui.   2. Cree
    Indians – Health and hygiene – Quebec (Province) – Whapmagoostui.
    3. Cree philosophy.   4. Health attitudes.   I. Title.

    E99.C88A333 2000   306'.089'973   C00-930395-2

University of Toronto Press acknowledges the financial assistance to its
publishing program of the Canada Council for the Arts and the Ontario Arts
Council.

This book has been published with the help of a grant from the Humanities
and Social Sciences Federation of Canada, using funds provided by the
Social Sciences and Humanities Research Council of Canada.

University of Toronto Press acknowledges the financial support for its publishing activities of the Government of Canada through the Book Publishing
Industry Development Program (BPIDP).

Contents

Acknowledgments

Providence, it seems, has played a large part in the preparation of this book. While the word suggests divine intervention, I would prefer to think of the interventions during the writing of this book as unconditionally divine but also (as far as I am aware) without any particular influences of higher forces, benevolent or otherwise. The benevolence of nature is another matter entirely. I had the good fortune to spend an entire winter as a guest at Providence, the name of a splendid property overlooking Island Creek, one of the many tributaries of the Choptank River on the Eastern Shore of Maryland. I could never have predicted that I would winter with the very same families of geese that fly above Whapmagoostui every year as they travel to and from their northern nesting grounds. And yet there I was with the geese and other migratory birds, in residence at Providence and working on the manuscript of this book in a wonderful cottage nestled at the edge of a forest of dogwood, and loblolly pine. The enchanting songbirds, bluebirds, owls, deer, and wintering Canada geese, ducks, and swans were delightful company. I offer a very special thank you to Mrs Harriet Critchlow, who provided me with a winter writer's residence.

Another form of 'divine' intervention must be acknowledged at the outset. A York University Faculty of Arts Fellowship awarded for the 1996–7 academic year provided me with the precious time needed to complete this book. Earlier assistance allowed me to conduct the research itself. I am particularly grateful to the National Health Research and Development Program (Health Canada grant #6606-3176-55), the McGill Centre for Northern Studies, the Social Science and Humanities Research Council of Canada, and the Max Bell Fellowship in Canadian Studies for providing all of the research support and graduate funding necessary to complete this project.

The kind people of Whapmagoostui have taught me so much over the years that simply saying 'thank you' seems inadequate. I hope this book does justice to all they have shared with me. I thank the Whapmagoostui First Nation Band Council, who on behalf of the community allowed me to conduct this project and all subsequent research with the people of Great Whale. *Ch'nskuu-midn.* I also thank the Cree Regional Board of Health and Social Services for supporting this project from its very inception.

I would like to take a moment to thank one person without whom this project would simply not have come to be. Emily Masty, MEd – mother, daughter, teacher, band councillor, and school principal – is a cherished friend and mentor. She is also, I hasten to add, the person who is most responsible for the onerous task of translating the words of her peers and elders that appear in this text. Emily's superb translation skills, for this project and for the many others on which she continues to work, are making the words of the Cree people come alive in English with unprecedented clarity and acumen. On a more personal note, Emily was the one who made sure that I got home safely at night, that someone always started the skidoo if I could not, that I was picked up from the airport, and that I was always properly fed. I am grateful for the many hours of discussion, laughter, meals, movies, and games we have shared. It is truly an honour to know such an extraordinary person, and I look forward to more collaborative efforts – and camping trips – with this dear friend.

There is a list of people a decade long who have been vital to the success of this project. I would like to take this opportunity to specifically thank Margaret Lock, Lisa M. Mitchell, Pamela Wakewich, Margaret Critchlow-Rodman, J. Teresa Holmes, Colin Scott, Dr Elizabeth Robinson, Helen Bobbish, and Joel Minion for their years of support, insight, and thoughtful commentary on this and other works. At University of Toronto Press, I thank Siobhan McMenemy for her wonderful assistance in the editorial process and the anonymous reviewers for their fine and instructive reading of this manuscript. In Whapmagoostui, I thank Emily Petagumskum for her excellent translation work. I also thank the entire Masty family (and especially Emily, Elizabeth, Susan, and Vera), Marianne and Tom Martin, Lisa Petagumskum, Arlene George, and Maggie Mamianskum and their respective families for making me feel at home from the moment I arrived. Most importantly, I thank all of the people who generously and patiently agreed to talk with me.

Thank you, Archie, for your timely gift of patience. *Chiisa ch'hiitn.* Finally, I am forever grateful to my parents and sisters for their unquestioning confidence in me and my seemingly circuitous path in life. I offer this book to them and dedicate it to my precious little daughter, Sophie Jeanne. Providence, indeed.

'BEING ALIVE WELL'

Chapter 1

'If the land is not healthy then how can we be?'[1]

Health, Bodies, and Resistance

'If the land is not healthy then how can we be?' No words can summarize more succinctly the essence of what it means to be healthy for the Whapmagoostui Cree.[2] The mention of land and its condition signals a broadened perspective on health that permeates not just one elder Cree man's words but the outlook of this entire book. Shaking loose any suppositions of a natural or universal definition of health, I take as a given that health is interpreted, idealized, and enacted in various ways. In other words, experiences and understandings of health and well-being are always historically and culturally mediated (Crawford, 1994; Litva & Eyles, 1994; Saltonstall, 1993). Indeed, from a Cree perspective, health has as much to do with social relations, land, and cultural identity as it does with individual physiology.

I begin with a modest assertion: health is never simply a neutral, biological category. Rather, from an anthropological perspective, I see 'health' as a complex, dynamic process, not as a baseline standard of biomedical or epidemiological normalcy. Furthermore, all definitions of health (including my own) are laden with ideological nuances and can never be separated from cultural norms and values, regardless of how the latter are played out in our everyday lives (Crawford, 1985; A. Young, 1980, 1982). I will explain what I mean by this over the next few pages, in which I highlight the key components of my general thesis on health. I will then devote the rest of this book to a discussion of what 'health' means in the Cree context. That context is incomplete without a broader knowledge of the history and contemporary circumstances of the Whapmagoostui Cree Nation, the people who now live along the Great Whale River in northern Quebec. In sum, this is first and foremost a book about the Whapmagoostui Cree and their concepts of health. Those concepts are inseparable from a particular socio-political reality and link the local biolog(ies) of a small population of adult Cree men and women with the larger themes of health and body politics (cf. Lock, 1993).

Some speak about how we have 'become obsessed with health' (McKnight, 1986: 77). That obsession, however, is not with a universal, knowable entity but rather with a particular cultural ideal. The obsession with which those in industrialized societies are most familiar is closely linked to particular ideals of bodily fitness and longevity. However, these two prominent characteristics of 'health' may or may not have anything to do with physiological wellness. Fitness and longevity speak more directly to an array of embodied symbols and dense metaphors peculiar to an individualistic, industrialized, modern world (Armstrong, 1983; Comaroff, 1985a; Worsley, 1982; Crawford, 1985, 1994; Lupton, 1995). Regardless of the result – whether trim or not, whether thirty or ninety – the prevailing image of our 'obsession' is that of a disease-free, fit, and youthful body (Lupton, 1995). More specifically, as Crawford succinctly states, 'The biomedical definition of the self is encoded as a cultural program with health as its personal, medical, and political objective' (1985: 63).

I am not suggesting that physiological wellness is an undesirable or unattainable goal. I *am* suggesting that this 'obsession' is important to note for a variety of reasons. First, these prevailing ideals of health exemplify the ways in which individuals embody and enact particular societal norms and values. Second, this dominant model of health so thoroughly permeates health discourse that it must be identified and marked as partial – that is, as both biased and incomplete. Too often health is presumed to be a natural category against which one can then determine a relative degree of nonhealth. Too often, as well, we presume universal ideals of bodily comportment and confuse or conflate them with similarly unrealistic ideas about some universally knowable standard of health. As Manning and Fabrega explain, 'The framework of Western biology and its concepts of function, structure, and performance are believed to order and constrain abilities located in or derived from the human body. Acceptance of what are assumed to be invariant and fundamental givens within the biological paradigm has created a cultural blindness, which can be the source of errors in [social scientific] analyses' (1973: 256).

Focusing specifically on anthropological writings, I have found that the ubiquitous conceptual link between health and disease predominates in the literature.[3] In the realms of ecological, political economic, and symbolic analysis, 'health' is rarely taken as the problematic. Rather, health is determined in proportion to a relative absence of disease, be it through the availability of medical services, the relative distribution of pathological environments, or population norms and standards (e.g., Dunn, 1968; McElroy & Townsend, 1985; McElroy, 1990; Frenk et al., 1991; Baer, 1986; Navarro, 1980; Kelman, 1980; Nichter, 1989; Wall, 1988; Ngubane, 1977; Janzen, 1981; Manning and Fabrega, 1973).[4] Even works that richly detail the cultural construction of health all too often do so in relation to illness or the healing process (Wall, 1988; Ngubane, 1977; Janzen, 1981; Manning and Fabrega, 1973).

What I attempt to do here is overcome the 'invariant and fundamental givens' of biomedical health. Health, as Saltonstall aptly summarizes, 'is not a universal fact, but is a constituted social reality, constructed through the medium of the body using the raw materials of social meaning and symbol' (1993: 12). Thus, health is neither a category nor an entity that can be known universally or against which one can determine the degree of nonhealth. Health is not readily subsumed or defined through health-seeking behaviours, health regulations, health promotion, or for that matter the absence of disease.[5] Similarly, population indicators provide little insight into the cultural determinants of health – except perhaps in a Foucauldian sense, as the imprint of regulatory norms. A pathology-oriented perspective obscures the grounded, conscious maintenance of health ideals – systems that are rooted in cultural norms and values and that may extend beyond the state of the physical body (Janzen, 1981). We must, in other words, attempt to rethink – rather than be constrained by – the framework of Western biology.

Furthermore, if we limit our study to the symbolic valuations of health, we may lose the historical, social, economic, and political influences that necessarily inform that (corpo)reality (Alexander, 1990). Recent studies of health have begun to problematize the rationale of a universal body and the construction of normalcy in health. In doing so, they are moving us beyond symbolic analyses toward a critical study of what health means. In particular, the body is increasingly becoming a central locus of inquiry as we pay closer attention to the embodiment of socio-political forces in studies of health. Buttressed by French social theorists such as Canguilhem, Foucault, and Bourdieu, anthropologists and sociologists are beginning to substantively rethink the theoretical and social boundaries of health. In particular, Canguilhem's *The Normal and the Pathological* (1989 [1966]) laid the foundation for French social theorists' ruminations on the connections between state power, the health of populations, and the body (Foucault, 1975, 1980, 1989). Through these and other works we are making new connections between the body in health (or illness) and the ways that people live, enact, or resist their social realities (Comaroff, 1985a, b; Lock, 1993; Lupton, 1995). We are, in other words, 'looking anew at the relations among biology, knowledge production and cultural context, trying to capture the imprint of social forces ... [and, by] documenting resistance to ideologies of social control [we are] learning how different practices change modes of knowing and conceptions of the self' (Lindenbaum and Lock 1993: xiv).

This brings us right back to the biomedical paradigm and its implications for the dominant model of health discussed above. The clearest connection between biology, knowledge production, and cultural context is found in the work of Robert Crawford (1980, 1985, 1994), who has written extensively on the cultural construction of health in North America. Crawford has found that the biomedical ideal of biological fitness is inseparable from the societal norms and values of individualism and control, which are defined together as 'health.' A biomedical concept of health permeates and is literally embodied in what people define as their own sense of well-being, so that values such as self-discipline, self-denial, control and will power are woven through – and impossible to disentangle from – interpretations of health. Ideas of health are so much a part of a 'commonsense' understanding of self that social norms and values such as individualism and control are seemingly inseparable from biomedical ideals of biological fitness (Crawford, 1985; Lupton, 1995). Health is increasingly subsumed within a rhetoric of control.

Again using Crawford's work as our baseline, let us now consider another aspect of this interpretation of health. What are the implications of health if it is forever tied to a host of societal prerogatives? If health is equated with control, can it then also somehow be restrictive and constraining? In other words, is a 'healthy' lifestyle one that is circumscribed by a particular and limited range of (what is constituted as) normal? Das (1990) would argue exactly this point. In her view, a presumed standard of biomedical, individuated fitness means far more than physiological wellness and constitutes a 'repressive ideology of health.' Measured in physiological terms, health and normalcy are one and the same, with vast implications for those who deviate from this norm (Crawford, 1994). When we root health in ideology, we are formulating it as equivalent to a prescribed standard of normalcy and establishing it as part of the routines of everyday life (Foucault, 1980; Armstrong, 1983; cf. Comaroff, 1985a). According to these standards, the state of being healthy constrains the individual to a proscribed biological and social morality, and this casts those who do not conform in strong relief against the chiselled backdrop of a naturalized conceptualization of health (Crawford, 1994).[6] With words that evoke the spirit of Foucault, Lupton describes this process of normalization: 'Every individual is now involved in observing, imposing and enforcing the regulations of public health, particularly through techniques of self-surveillance

and bodily control encouraged by the imperatives of health promotion' (Lupton, 1995: 76).[7]

A repressive ideology of health offers little more than a bleak
and restrictive exploration of the embodiment of state power. Das
(1990), Comaroff (1985a,b), and B. Turner (1985) all argue that
this perspective far too narrowly defines the individual as something akin to an involuntary player shaped according to the bid-
ding of the State. Is health always related to restrictive forms of
power, or can it equally be related to the processes of resistance
(Das 1990)? In his analysis of health, Crawford, too, deplores this
sort of passive compliance, arguing that 'as long as the dominant
metaphors of health connote control, we lend our participation
to a regime of disciplinary power and to the self-discipline on
which it relies, to a self-regulating, contained selfhood that nar-
rows our identities to that which is compatible with various insti-
tutional, corporate and bureaucratic agendas' (1994: 1364).

Das (1990) similarly contends that while the individual is
defined by society, one may also resist that definition. It follows
that health must be redefined in order to account for that resistance. Das views health from within a liberating paradigm, not
from one that – by an implicit adherence to processes of normalization – perpetuates a model of regulative power. According to
Das, the problem is that these (latter) 'ideologies of health may
rob one of one's personhood and one's place in society' (1990:
45). Crawford (1985) and Lupton (1995), too, have found pock-
ets of resistance permeating those regulative ideals of health.
Both suggest that the very processes which are restrictive can
alternatively be viewed as forms of release or (more broadly)
resistance. In other words, health as discipline and self-denial can
be viewed as liberating; individualistic conceptions of health,
while replete with hegemonic meanings, can at the same time be
appropriated in an attempt to counter perceived obstacles to
health and ultimately, identity (Lupton, 1995; Crawford, 1985).

Das (1990), Crawford (1985, 1994), and Lupton (1995) all provide ground-breaking arguments for the distancing of health
from illness. In so doing they shift the emphasis away from the
regulatory and normalizing models of health and situate health

simultaneously within the realm of the sentient individual and the domain of resistance. They also remind us that a proper social scientific study of health is part and parcel of the larger examination of how social forces are embodied. I will now take that discussion one step further. Rather than remain within the dominant health paradigm – either as passive or active participant – I now move to a different position using the Cree example. I take as a given that health and, more specifically, health ideals are rooted in cultural norms and values that permeate and define – yet extend beyond – the state of the physical body. Indeed, among the Whapmagoostui Cree the concept of health – *miyupimaatisiiun* – ultimately transcends the individual, and as part of the realm of 'being Cree' is linked to a larger strategy of cultural assertion and resistance in a dynamic balancing of power between the State, the disenfranchised group, and the individual.

In other words, health is political. By this I mean that health takes on a particular, and particularly charged, meaning when understood within its historical, cultural, and social context. Furthermore, for the Cree, health is inseparable from 'being Cree.' 'Being Cree,' in turn, is a process of identification, a marker of self-in-the-world that is forever located within a text of historical accountings, land, and the production and interpretation of specific and distinctive beliefs and activities. I do not purport that there is one definitive way to 'be Cree' (or to be healthy, for that matter); nor am I suggesting that culture can be bound or reproduced either in life or in text. There is no question that the context and parameters of health shift with time and place. It is extremely important to note, however, that *miyupimaatisiiun*, as it was described to me, offers a means of making sense of the profoundly vital links between 'health,' politics, and Cree identity.

Context and Content

For the Cree of Whapmagoostui, a sense of 'health' – or of 'being Cree,' for that matter – cannot be understood outside the context of colonial and neo-colonial relations in Canada. Indigenous Canadians – Indian, Inuit, or Métis – continue to live with the effects of displacement, discriminatory legislation, failed attempts at assimilation, forced religious conversion, and pervasive racism. Some communities and individuals have fared better than others, and without doubt a growing number of success stories are able to be told. Whapmagoostui has its own stories of successes and failures, some originating from within the community, and some not.

The recent possibility that their homeland and hunting grounds may be eradicated stands today as one of the greatest possible failures imposed on the Whapmagoostui Cree. In 1989 the Quebec provincial government announced that a massive hydro-electric project would be built on the Great Whale River. That announcement rekindled old animosities and became the unwelcome centrepiece in a story that few wanted to either hear or tell. Yet this new threat to the Eastern Cree was not entirely unexpected or unfamiliar. Twenty years earlier the village of Chisasibi, about 200 kilometres to the south, had lost a battle against a similar hydro-electric project. Long before that, Europeans had come to this northern region in search of minerals, furs, and (the most lucrative local resource in the 1800s) whale oil. Over the last 300 years, prospectors, fur traders, cartographers, whalers, post managers, missionaries, and (later) nurses, hospital ships, pilots, biologists, anthropologists, and teachers, and even the armed forces, have left their mark on the land and its people. I mention these earlier visitors to suggest the depth and complexity of relations between outsiders and the people of the Great Whale River region. The hydro-electric project was slated to become yet another imposition from 'the south' – another chapter in the long and all too often predictable history of native/ non-native relations. A far too familiar historical pattern was shattered, however, when the project was defeated six hard-fought years after it was announced. The project and its defeat are necessarily part of this story of health, though not the central focus of the book. The events that surrounded the project constitute something of a continuous 'white noise' – an incessant reminder of the asymmetrical power balance between Native Canadians and the nation-state.[8]

In telling this story I am quite particular in my use of specific terms such as 'Cree,' 'Native Canadian,' 'nation-state,' and 'white-man.' Regardless of the volumes that have been written on the fluidity, heterogeneity, and complexity of such categories, few in Whapmagoostui have considered an alternative to the word 'whiteman' (*waamstikuushiiu*) – or 'Indian,' for that matter. Deal-ings with the world beyond Whapmagoostui take place at many levels and in a multiplicity of forms, yet the disaffinity felt toward the world outside Whapmagoostui is anything but diverse. There is a particular, homogeneous 'other' – an entity, if not an individ-ual *per se*, that is spoken of as *waamstikuushiiu* or 'whiteman.' That entity has continued to remove indigenous peoples to a smaller and smaller space on the political, economic, social, *and* geo-graphic maps of Canada. The term *waamstikuushiiu* encapsulates and concretizes the remembered and recurring iniquities so familiar to generations of Cree people (cf. Tsing, 1993). Ulti-mately, to understand what 'health' means to the Cree is to understand something of that process.

The northern Cree have been faced with, have challenged, and have sometimes wholeheartedly embraced many, many changes over the past two centuries, and in the past four decades in partic-ular. Satellite dishes, fax machines, computers, and web sites are as much a part of northern living as skidoos, rifles, and the ubiq-uitous Northern Stores (formerly, the Hudson's Bay Company posts). Men and women who spent most of their years travelling and working in the bush now see their children and grandchil-dren watching satellite television, playing team hockey, and surf-ing the Internet as readily as they might hunt caribou or pluck geese. Fifty years ago a large hospital ship would sail around Hud-son Bay, stopping at each post once a year to X-ray the chest of each and every native person. Those who showed any signs of tuberculosis, regardless of age, were shipped south to sanatoria for months or years at a time. Less than fifty years ago virtually all births took place in the bush with the assistance of an older, expe-rienced Cree midwife. Today, a modern clinic serves all of the basic medical needs of the community, although all pregnant women are still evacuated weeks before their due date to give birth at the one regional hospital, in Chisasibi; less often they are sent even further south to either Val d'Or or Montreal. All must leave the community to give birth, although some do admit that the required and often burdensome trip allows them to indulge in shopping at stores that simply do not exist in the North.

Along with the clinic have come a bright new school, a day care centre, and an indoor hockey arena. The village also boasts modern houses, although some complain they are getting sick living in those houses and that there are simply not enough homes – good or bad – for the rapidly growing community. Teenagers and young adults who are not employed, or who do not play sports or hunt on a regular basis, complain of being terribly bored; all too often they turn to alcohol and drugs as a diversion from everyday life. Unemployment compounds the problems faced by young and old alike. There have been vast changes, in other words, in a very short period of time, with both positive and negative effects.

With the availability of print and electronic media, with a provincial Cree leadership, and with regular plane travel into and out of the community, the horizons of the Cree world have expanded significantly over the past few years. The people of Whapmagoostui are now much less isolated from the greater indigenous Canadian reality; they are connected not only to the rest of the Eastern Cree nation, but also to the Cree of western Canada and to other indigenous nations across North and South America and around the world. One event in particular resonated deeply with the people of Whapmagoostui: the Oka Crisis – a prolonged armed struggle that erupted in 1990 when a Quebec municipality near Montreal unilaterally decided to turn Mohawk burial grounds and forest lands into a golf course – became a watershed event that led to a new era of indigenous self-awareness and strength right across Canada. During the long, hot summer of 1990, the ponytails and bandannas sported by the Mohawk men and seen every night on the evening news were equally as evident hundreds of kilometres away on the teenagers of Whapmagoostui. This was a statement of new connections and even greater political awakenings among the Cree youth – youth who were already engaging in their own community's battle to keep their lands intact.

Cultural distinctiveness and sovereign title to land take on additional meaning when proclaimed in Quebec. Throughout the 1990s the Quebec nationalists' struggle for independence from Canada loomed close to the surface of any debate around aboriginal rights. Quebec's long-standing threat to separate from the rest of Canada, and the recent assertion by the Quebec government that the entire province would be governed as sovereign property, have been met head on by the provincial Cree leadership. Armed with the Cree-Naskapi Act, the Cree leadership continues to remind the provincial government that the Cree are a self-governing body on lands that are, by earlier agreement, removed from sovereigntist claims. The Cree people will not allow their lands to be subsumed within a separate Quebec. They are also fully aware of the irony of the sovereigntist claims, given their own struggle for political and economic autonomy.

Through all the changes, influences, and threats, each generation continues to learn, embody, and envision the myriad ways of being Cree. For some, being Cree means a life of trapping, fishing, and hunting; for others, it means running a wholly Cree-owned logging company, gas station, or video store. For some, being Cree includes adopting the ways of the Anglican or evangelical Christian church; for others, native spirituality is the truest and only form of religious expression; for still others, any overt religious affiliation is simply more evidence of oppression and assimilation. There is no one way to 'be Cree' – there is no single way to live or express oneself as a Cree person.

Modern native identities are forged in the heat of colonial and neocolonial realities. For this reason, too, we cannot simply speak of any sort of decontextualized 'Cree culture.' Yet the Cree themselves can readily point to what they consider essential to what it means to be a Cree person. These are issues of identity, issues that are rooted in a sense of culture but that are not defined as culture per se. People in Whapmagoostui are trying to pay their bills, keep food on the table, and maintain important and consequential links to their cultural past, present, and future. It is the very banality of this sense of being Cree that makes these things all the more potent. In reference to artistic production, Turner Strong and Van Winkle speak of essentialist discourse as the 'tragically necessary condition for the continued survival and vitality of many individuals and communities' (1996: 565). I agree, but caution that there is a difference between native authors and artists who define their art in part as a rage against domination, and the lives of people far removed from such esoterica. What I find so profoundly important in this study of health is the way in which identities are defined through a sense of things rooted in the joys and struggles of daily living. This is not simply a romantic heralding of an irretrievable past. These are people recounting the stories of their lives and the lives of their parents and grandparents – stories that continue to resonate for the Cree of Whapmagoostui. The sincerity of these histories, accompanied by increasing difficulties in people's ability to 'be healthy,' lends such strength to their stories that they can only be understood in the context of identity, power, and resistance.

This is not a book about disease or illness. There is a tremendously broad literature devoted to the morbidity and mortality of indigenous populations (e.g., Waldram, Herring, and Young, 1995; T.K. Young, 1988a). Accidental and suicidal deaths, drug- and alcohol-related illnesses, infectious diseases, and chronic diseases such as diabetes mellitus and cancer are all found – sometimes in disproportionate number – in native communities across Canada. Whapmagoostui is not immune to these problems. But to dwell on disease statistics in this study of health would be to view indigenous communities far too narrowly as somehow always being either sick or out of control (Waldram, Herring, and Young, 1995). When speaking about health, and in particular Cree health, the first step to understanding its various meanings is to not confuse disease with the study of health.

'Being Alive Well'

For the Cree there is no word that translates into English as 'health.' The most apt phrase is *miyupimaatisiiun* or, as I translate it, 'being alive well.' 'Being alive well' constitutes what one may describe as being healthy; yet it is less determined by bodily functions than by the practices of daily living and by the balance of human relationships intrinsic to Cree lifestyles. 'Being alive well' means that one is able to hunt, to pursue traditional activities, to eat the right foods, and (not surprisingly, given the harsh northern winters) to keep warm. This is above all a matter of quality of life. That quality of life is linked, in turn, to political and social phenomena that are as much a part of the contemporary Cree world as are the exigencies of 'being alive well' (see also Lacasse, 1982; Kistabish, 1982; Meehan, 1982).

In this book I present and explain the symbols and meanings of 'being alive well' for the Whapmagoostui Cree adults as they were described to me.[9] 'Being alive well' speaks to ideals that can only be enacted through what is immediately understood as 'being Cree'; as such, it is a focal point around which the adult Cree articulate their sense of being and belonging. I was troubled at first by the homogeneity that permeated the stories I was hearing. For example, why when I asked about 'health' were people always talking to me about the land, the animals, and their lives in the bush? And why was there such similarity between these stories? Where were the inconsistencies, the nodes of difference? Finally I began to listen more carefully and to hear what the stories were telling me. Instead of teasing out anomalies, I began to ask myself why the stories I was being told were so consistently similar.

In the next chapter I offer a fairly extensive history of the people and the region; in that process, I examine the accommodations the Cree have made to European economic and political rule. I then move to the core of this book: descriptions of the idealized and lived experiences of 'being alive well.' These descriptions exemplify distinctive Cree practices, since 'being alive well' has everything to do with a particular way of 'being Cree.' Given the context in which one can or cannot 'be Cree,' it is hardly surprising that it is through 'being alive well' that we see an articulation of physical, moral, political, and social forces that coalesce into a sense of Cree health, identity, and ultimately dissent.

Working and Living in Whapmagoostui

A teenager from Whapmagoostui asked me recently why I had chosen to speak over the years only with the adults of the community. I told her that I felt the younger adults, teens, and children deserve an entirely separate focus, since the influences on them and the choices they will have differ so radically from those of their parents' and grandparents' generations (cf. Masty, 1995). I still believe this to be true; but in retrospect I also feel that this was a less than adequate response. This inadequacy, however, is related more to my ambivalence about my role as an anthropologist in an indigenous community than to the specifics of the research she was suggesting. The relationship between anthropologists and native communities in Canada is tenuous at best. What right do I have to walk, however cautiously, in the footsteps of those who for so long simply reproduced the colonial order? I continue to struggle with this question, wondering how much I am contributing to a new order and how much I am inadvertently reproducing an older one.

In a time when voices and perspectives are contested, resisted, deconstructed, and reconstructed, I do not pretend to speak *for* the Whapmagoostui people. That is neither my place nor my intent. I had an opportunity to speak *with* the people, and they in turn spoke with me. I offer my representation of what people told me about themselves and about their sense of health. 'You have a perspective, a way of interpreting our stories,' a Cree friend told me. 'It is not the only perspective, but it is just as valid as any of ours.' Through talks with members of the community, I see how our various interpretations add to the ongoing discussions of aboriginal issues. I have situated my interpretation within the context of anthropology, and hence must reconcile the animosity felt by some toward the discipline. It is comforting, at least, to know that the people of Whapmagoostui have given me the opportunity and permission to reflect on their words, their thoughts, and their actions.

I began the process of writing this book by rereading my original field notes, searching through them for those long-forgotten initial sensations of arriving in a community that has since become part of my life. The hours spent reading those early journals kindled various memories – the trepidation of a young anthropologist, the excitement of bush camp, first feasts, and even first Skidoo rides, along with all of the frustrations that are part of living in any new place before both friendships and work fill the emotional and temporal hollows. My anxieties, too, were dredged up – I had forgotten just how carefully I had to avoid those who drank, being sure to lock my doors at night and not to step out too early on weekend mornings, in case I encountered a reveller still on his way home.

I was also starkly reminded of how conscious I was of being single, white, and female in Whapmagoostui.[10] Being 'white,' yet living and circulating exclusively within the Cree community, I was certainly not one of the 'whites' who lived 'up the hill'[11] from the Cree; yet neither was I Cree. Those who knew me only by sight referred to me simply as *wamistikushiiu'ishgaw*, generic 'white woman.' Later I came to be known as 'the woman with the red hair'; but soon enough, and far more commonly, I became just 'Nahim,' a Cree nickname for Naomi. Searching through the Cree lexicon book one day, I came across the Cree word for Jewish person. 'That's what I am,' I told my companion, 'I'm *chuu'iiy-iyu*.' My friend explained that I was hence technically not *wamistikushiiu'ishgaw*, regardless of my skin colour. I must admit to feeling some relief when I learned of this, as if a burden of history had somehow been removed from my shoulders. The stories we then traded about racism and genocide reminded me of other burdens, but at least these we could share.

As a woman, my activities were more restricted yet somehow also freer. I could not readily join the men on hunting excursions, but as a professional researcher I could sit and converse with both men and women without threatening either group. It was highly unlikely, however, that a man would choose to work as my translator. Male pride was not the issue here, so much as the embarrassment our working together might cause for either that man or myself. I learned quickly enough how much teasing and joking goes on as part of everyday life in Whapmagoostui – and how difficult gossip is to live down in such a small community. I eventually did find two excellent translators to assist me with the formal interviews. Both were women.

Being single posed another set of problems. When I first arrived in Whapmagoostui, I was old enough to have both husband and children but had neither; thus, my status as an adult was put into question. My early skills in the bush also suggested anything but adult status, single or otherwise. I was indeed a child in my knowledge and abilities when plucking geese, and starting a fire, and gathering and laying a tent's carpet of fir boughs. I am pleased that after years of guidance, I have become far more proficient (though hardly an expert) in the necessary bush skills. In those early years I was alternatively a guest, a family member, a child, an adult, a novice, and, in rare instances, an expert. I was laughed at during my early, feeble attempts to speak Cree, and chided when I hurried and tried to pluck more than one goose feather at a time; yet I was also called upon for first aid assistance, for certain cooking skills when needed, and for making sense of some unusual English expressions. Single, 'white,' and female separately and together affected the ways in which my social activities and my work were defined. It would be naïve to think otherwise.

A Note on Anonymity

The place is real, and Whapmagoostui is its real name. Beyond that, and with only one exception, I conceal the identity of the people who so generously shared their time and stories with me. This is a terrible disservice to those individuals, since these narratives tell of *their* lives and *their* histories. Bound by the rules that govern the ethical conduct of research, however, I promised to protect the anonymity of all those who agreed to talk with me before the first interview ever began. I am obliged to the community and the larger readership to forego the nuances that come with identity for the larger narrative that is told in the combination of these stories.

Initials and pseudonyms do not sit well with me. They presume either secrecy or simulation, as though I am really telling another's story entirely. Thus when I do quote directly from interviews or discussions, the translated words are presented here in italics, but with no referent other than the occasional notation indicating whether the speaker is a man or a woman.

Chapter 2

The Whapmagoostui *Iyiyuu'ch*

At some point – perhaps when the village became a permanent site, or when the schools were opened and children were required to stay at the post for longer periods of time, or when anthropologists arrived and began recording and writing about the people living in their summer residence, or perhaps even more recently, when Great Whale divided officially into Whapmagoostui and Kuujjuarapik – the history of the Cree and the history of the village began to coalesce into virtually interchangeable histories. Today we talk about the approximately 600 people *from* Whapmagoostui, not always differentiating between those who live there all the time and those who only appear twice a year from their hunting grounds or trap lines.[1] We also talk about the Cree Nation of Whapmagoostui – a political entity and part of the combined eastern James Bay Cree First Nation – and no longer about the northern hunters, a northern Algonquian band, or even just simply the people of the region.

Approximately 1400 kilometres north of Montreal, the immense, winding Great Whale River flows into Hudson Bay. At the mouth of the Great Whale, on a spit of land between the river and the enormous bay, on the edge of the vast subarctic expanse, is the village of Whapmagoostui. Whapmagoostui is situated on the taïga, a transitional zone between boreal forest and the treeless tundra. Inland is the characteristic panorama of tamarack, spruce, pine, birch, and willow trees, an array of hardy plants and low shrubs, and carpets of spongy moss. In contrast, the Hudson

Bay shoreline is virtually barren; fierce northerly winds blow inland and discourage all but the most robust plants from taking root among the weather-smoothed rock beds and ponds. Although you have to bend low to find it, the crevices of these rocks yield a surprisingly rich summer harvest. In among the moss and the diminutive arctic flowers are blueberries, cranberries, bakeapple berries, blackberries, and (small leaf) Labrador tea, the latter collected and stored for use as a wonderfully soothing and aromatic tonic. On the rocks grows a hard black lichen that crunches underfoot. I was told many times how that lichen was boiled into a miserably thin porridge when times were especially hard and the choice was to eat it or starve.

There are still no roads this far north into Quebec. If remoteness is a question of ease of access, then Whapmagoostui remains a remote village. The community still relies on air transport for its mail and all its store-bought foods. That reliance is often frustrated by the vicissitudes of nature and politics.[2] With no radar tower because of complicated disputes surrounding its construction, and with either fog so dense or storms so violent that no plane can land with only visual instrumentation, days can go by with nothing and no one coming in or going out. In the few months of the year when the waterways are accessible, large supply boats enter Hudson Bay loaded down with such things as the annual store of fuel, construction equipment and materials, trucks, Skidoos, and dry goods for the village's three general stores.[3]

In some ways, then, Whapmagoostui remains remote from the major cities of Quebec and Canada. Yet if we think of the various other means by which we traverse distance today, Whapmagoostui is neither remote nor isolated. Telephones and fax machines are readily available and heavily used; indeed, they are an indispensable part of life throughout the Canadian North. For many years satellite dishes were operated by the single 'social club' (i.e., bar) in town, drawing in a range of television stations, which were then relayed to the houses in the community. Today many homes have individual satellite dishes. There are also at least four radio stations available, although many adults listen primarily to the one Cree-language radio. More recently, a class of high school students and

their computer teacher have created an Internet home page linking them not only to the James Bay Cree Nation home page but
to the entire world of cybercommunication (www.web.apc.org/
~badabin/home.htm). Finally, and most importantly, if we think
of Whapmagoostui as a centre – as a place and a region where people are born and live their entire lives, as a place that a world
begins *at* and extends *from*, not as a place where the world 'ends' –
then it is anything but remote.

There are nine eastern Cree communities, all part of the James
Bay Cree Nation. Each of these settlements – the original eight
plus the recently established ninth, Oujé-Bougamou – is now a
nation in itself as well as a separate component of the larger
James Bay Cree Nation. The flag that flies atop the Whapmagoostui First Nation band office building signals the recent shift in
designation from band to village to nation. The Whapmagoostui
Cree First Nation flag depicts the most common three animals
hunted in this region: goose, caribou, and bear. That emblem,
which one sees emblazoned on T-shirts, caps, and official letter-
head, marks the recent changes in the practical and conceptual
organization of this community. This is a nation among nations.

The Space of the Nation

'Leave us alone!' Elizabeth calls into the sky, trying to shout down
the *thwack-thwack* of a helicopter that has suddenly broken the
morning calm at her family's spring goose camp. Just 20 kilometres north of the village and a few hundred metres from the frozen shoreline of Hudson Bay, Elizabeth and her sisters and their
families are settled in at their spring goose-hunting camp. The
last thing one expects to see or hear is an aircraft flying so low
overhead. Shaking her fist at the unwelcome sight, she adds,
'What do they want now? Don't they know they are going to scare
away the geese?' A Hydro-Quebec survey craft is making yet
another tour of a planned turbine site. But this is hunting space,
and the helicopter is an especially hostile reminder of what Elizabeth and the rest of the community are fighting against in their
bid to halt the Great Whale River hydro-electric project.

Goose camp is a twice-annual hunting event that coincides with the spring and fall migration of Canada geese. It has long been a cherished time for the Cree of northern Quebec. Entire families head out to their respective camps, and most spend the better part of two weeks living off the land, harvesting and feasting on this highly valued food (see also C. Scott, 1983, 1989b). Jobs at the band office, school, store, or garage are put on hold when the geese are flying. Spring and fall goose breaks turn the village into a virtual ghost town. Men of all ages will go out in smaller groups to hunt or fish at other times of the year, but goose break involves everyone – as children, parents, and grandparents head out to camps that stretch for kilometres to the north and south of the Great Whale River. Preparations for hunting camp – buying and readying tents, guns, and equipment – begin months before the actual departure, as people watch the weather patterns, recall past years, and debate whether the season will be a good one.

In some ways the village and the bush are completely separate, each defined by what the other is not. In other ways, village and bush life are integrated – just as some of the conveniences and foods associated with village life have been integrated into camp life, so too have camp activities been implanted in village routines. This is especially true near the end of goose-hunting season, when the women use the many tipis (*miichuap*) dotting the village as places for plucking and preparing the geese that have been brought home. The tipis are also used to smoke caribou hides and to cook or dry other meats. They are also, when a low fire is burning, a wonderful place to relax and visit. The village and the bush are two parts of the larger whole of life here. However often people speak about the ruinous effects of village life – of the boredom and the alcohol and the store-bought foods – they continue to negotiate the routines, events, and commodities of both the village and the bush.

My exploration of 'health' led me directly into that intermediate terrain as people shared with me their thoughts about what it means to live well, to be 'healthy' as a Cree person. This is a space that is filled with both tension and contentment, with both contradictions and consistencies as people establish connections between their personal and collective past, present, and future. 'Health,' as I finally came to learn, has everything to do with how one negotiates that terrain, and how people reconcile their sense of themselves as *Iyiyuu'ch*, as Cree people. A sense of health is ultimately rooted in what it means to 'be Cree,' and being Cree has everything to do with connections to the land and to a rich and complex past. I move, then, to an exploration of that past, beginning with a story from one elder woman's history that carries us back into the history of the Whapmagoostui *Iyiyuu'ch*, the people.

Well, ever since I remember, there was so little of everything, there wasn't very much of anything. That was while my father was raising us. Since then, I have already seen how hard it is to survive. I had two brothers who did the hunting for the family. It was so hard sometimes when it was difficult for them to kill something for the family. And most of the time we were always so hungry, that was the time they didn't have much luck hunting. But still we wouldn't come to the trading post for a whole year, and still we survived. Still we survived, we only ate the animals that they killed, we ate fish. A couple of times we weren't so lucky but sometimes we were lucky. Sometimes it seemed like it was easy for them to kill something when they were lucky. Even sometimes when we were not lucky, but sometimes we got lucky. That's how life was. Sometimes it was so hard when there was hardly any food to eat. That was when they weren't lucky to kill anything. But we still made it through the year, because usually we started our journey in August and we would return to Great Whale River in July. We were so far away from here, that's how far we were, the rivers were going on the other side. That's where my father's hunting ground was. I guess we were at the farthest place of any other people. Even north of Lac Bienville – that's why they didn't bother to come to the trading post because it was so far from where we were. My two brothers – one of them is still alive – that's why they never bothered to come to the trading post because it was so far, where they were. They wouldn't even think about coming to the trading post, even if they didn't have any supplies; we didn't even use anything that runs itself [with a motor], because everything that we did, we walked. Everything we did was by walking, if we had to go somewhere else, we walked, we made all of our transportation. It seems so far, if a person knew exactly the place we were. So in the spring we would ... start our journey down to Great Whale River. We would start our journey in the spring after ice break. Imagine how far we were in the winter and we would start our journey after the ice broke. Well, sometimes it wasn't that bad, it wasn't so bad, that's how we made it through the year. Sometimes, I remember my father got so lucky, he usually killed a lot of otter. That's what he collected for fur, and mink and marten; there was hardly any beaver. There were quite a few mink, marten, and otter so that's what they caught in the winter. They would really have a lot of furs if they wanted to. Once we made it here, when my father sold his furs, after we would have some whiteman's food. They wouldn't have any work to do while they were here, there was never any work to do. There was never work around and that was the only time they would help themselves with their furs. That would be the only way to make some money when we returned here. We were only here for a while, once we were here, we were only here for a short while. We returned here in July – sometimes we would return at the end of June – and by the end of August we would start our journey back. That's when we headed back north and it's not like now. Many times, I realize, just watching how many furs they killed in a year, my two brothers and my father, and what kind of furs they had – marten, mink, and otter, just how little money they would have made from their furs ... When we were away for the whole year without going to the trading post, that's how life was ever since I remember it. That's how they made their living and survived through the years, even if they didn't go to the trading post. I don't think there were many people who stayed here [in Great Whale River] because most of the people were gone, that was when all the people were still alive, even when the ones who are not anymore. People in the past, they wouldn't stay here for anything – they would rather stay in the bush because that was the only way they could survive because they had to work hard to survive. But life is different right now – it seems the people get sick right now, the things they are using, the things we use right now, the things they are using, as the things we use right now, not like in the past, when the people were healthy and strong. That was before they started using whiteman's food. Most of the people spent their lifetime in the bush. And there were quite a few lakes where we got lucky with fish, even if we didn't eat caribou, even if they didn't kill anything else besides fish, we would get lucky with fish and that was how we would survive.

Recollecting the Past

The essence of what it means to be Cree, and the substantiation of the Cree people as a distinct cultural group, is grounded in the oral historical record and in the recollections of familial and individual pasts. As illustrated in the above story, the past emerges through a chronology of events, lives, and seasons of travel. These histories describe the activities of individuals; in their telling and retelling they also suffuse the modern Cree person with a particular sense of identity so that the past is not merely recorded in memory, but is at the same time part of how current identities are imagined and enacted. These images infuse the activities of daily living with profound meaning, so that 'the past as it is represented becomes embodied and thereby achieves its force as part of the living present' (Kapferer, 1989: 189; Shils, 1981).

As with other oral hunting cultures, Cree history is passed down through the generations mainly in the form of stories, and cultural artifacts such as clothing and tools. The tales in particular tell listeners how various individuals used their survival skills across vast territories and in a variety of situations. There is also a wealth of stories of ancient ancestors, of encounters with the supernatural world, and of how the Cree world and people came into being.[4]

Once there was a man long ago. He was a man who was recognized as a very successful hunter. As time went on, suddenly he was not getting anything at all no matter what he did and even though he was out hunting every day till night. Soon they were very hungry. One day as he was out hunting, he heard a group of children at play in the distance. He went where the voices were coming from. There he came upon a group of children who were sliding. He took off his snowshoes at the base of the trail where the children's sliding route was. He spoke to the children but they acted as if he was not there. Long time ago, when a person comes upon a camp of people, he would announce himself by saying, 'I am a visitor.' He said to the children, 'I am a visitor.' But the children did not respond. He thought to himself, 'The children are just too busy being children.' He went into the woods where he knew the dwellings were. He could tell that the people at the biggest dwelling were crushing and pounding the caribou bones to collect the fat by the sounds he heard. He was closer to a smaller dwelling and he poked his head in the dwelling. There were two groups of women on either side of the dwelling in the process of tanning caribou skins. He announced himself to them saying, 'I am a visitor.' The women did not respond. It was as if he was not there at all. They did not acknowledge his presence at all. He went to the biggest dwelling and announced himself again saying, 'I am a visitor.' Again, no one responded to him. He began to get suspicious – because he had powers. He entered the dwelling anyway and went straight for the back of the dwelling [which is the place of honour, and usually where guests are told to sit or sleep]. He sat himself between two men who were sitting there. The men were just sitting down to eat the boiled meat, cut from the caribou bones. No one seemed to notice his presence and no one spoke to him. The men he sat with were being served straight from the pot and onto their plates. The men all started to eat. Of course, he was the only one not eating because he had not been given any food to eat. He was desperate for something to eat, so he cut a piece of meat from one of the men beside him. When he had finished eating the first piece of meat, he cut another piece of meat from the other man on his other side and ate that meat. As each man got up to leave they each said the same thing: 'Could it be true what the children said when they said they felt the presence of someone or something?' Soon there was no one left in that dwelling. He went to the dwelling where the women were but there was no one in that dwelling either. He listened for the children but he did not hear them nor did he see anyone about. He got suspicious – for he had powers. He gathered up the bones and all the meat that he saw. He also gathered up all the caribou skins and put all these things in one place. There were huge platforms of meat and he took down all of those, too. He just gathered all the food he saw in one place. This is where I do not know how the story goes, whether he took some of the food with him back to his camp. He went back to his camp. I guess he was feeling well because he had eaten the meat he had stolen from them, so to speak. When got back to his camp, he started to become suspicious of what had happened to him. He did not realize yet that he had visited the camp of his spirit guide.[5] When he got back to his camp, he built a shaking tent. As soon as it was built and he went in, his spirit guide entered the shaking tent. He told his spirit guide what he had experienced. His spirit guide told him that it was them that he had visited. His spirit guide said, 'We were the ones who you saw. You did not kill the animals that you should have because we killed the animals that you should have killed. All the food that you saw at our camp, it will all be yours. It is rightfully yours because you should have killed all that food. You can have it for your own use and your children's.' That is exactly what he did. He moved camp to where all the food was. He stayed there and used all the food his spirit guide had killed. From that day on he did not have bad luck with his hunting again, it is told. From then on, he was successful with his hunting. I suppose his spirit guide in turn did not kill anything to eat! [laughs]

The spirit guides; the spirits that live under the waterfalls; the giants whose footsteps moulded the landscape; the Cree people's dealings with the Lady Spirit of the Caribou; the long months of travel, hunting, and fishing, or of starvation and death; and the negotiations with the Inuit and with European traders – all of these tell the history of the Cree and their land. A hilltop or wooded area may be named for someone who was born or died there, or for a special or supernatural event which took place on that spot. In other words, the history of the people and the history of the land do not simply correspond to each other – they are one and the same. These histories bend and flow with the contours of the land and rivers of this northern region. They are also bred in the bones, as impossible to disentangle from hills and portage sites as they are from the events that permeate peoples' daily lives today.

These histories endure through the generations as they are told and retold in stories and cautionary tales and replayed in overt practices. Some people tell the stories directly to their children and grandchildren; others borrow or buy recorded tapes made by a local elder, who is especially good at detail and tells a good story. In a realistic assessment of the changing times, one Whapmagoostui woman has taken it on herself to record and transcribe hundreds of histories of the people and the region, knowing that as the present generation of elders dies, their stories of entire lives lived on the land will die with them (Masty and Marshall, n.d.).

The histories of the Whapmagoostui people – however they are recounted and wherever they are told – are fundamental to our understanding of the relationship between identity and 'being alive well.' In telling the history of the Whapmagoostui *Iyiyuu'ch*, one could begin in any of a number of different places or times. I begin, arbitrarily, with how people distinguish themselves in relation to their parents' lives and livelihoods. That will bring us quickly to the history of 'contact,' and on up to the present day. This is by no means the only way to tell the story of the Cree people, and admittedly it relies far too heavily on an imposed order and chronology. Unfortunately, such a temporal ordering places events within a history that builds on expansion and development, and places the key players in Canadian northern history in a field of relations too often defined primarily by travellers' records and factors' diaries. Much of Cree history has been recorded in this way (by non-native authors) – as if it is synonymous with the history of contact. For example, early missionary and anthropological accounts provide written details of contact, and while they do offer some tremendous insights into the material culture of the mid-nineteenth century, they are written in the shadow of social evolutionary thought. Neither those accounts nor any others can capture the depth and extent of Cree history, a history that goes back further than when 'the animals and the people could still speak to one another.' The ordered chronology that I present here is a means for placing 'being alive well' in its social and historical context. I have spliced into this chapter a selection of histories told to me by some of the elders of Whapmagoostui in order to add some nuance and perspective to my somewhat drier account. With that framework in place, I will devote the next chapter to an explanation of 'being alive well.'

One day, my uncle discussed separating [from the rest of the family] to hunt somewhere else. He would take his whole family with him. My father did not try to stop him. When they had left, we also went somewhere else to hunt. That very first day we moved camp, it was the first time we ate it seemed. My father killed an otter and he also brought some ptarmigan. The days were longer now. My father said, 'I saw another set of otter tracks and I will follow them tomorrow. You will put fish lines in while I am gone.' There was a lake nearby that looked like good fishing there. 'You put the fish lines in,' he said to my mother. I had an older brother but he was not an adult yet. 'You go with our son when you set the fish lines in the water. I also sighted some trees that have been eaten by a porcupine and I want you to go walking around to see if you can find the porcupine,' he said to my mother. The rest of us younger children sat with my grandmother. Our grandmother was looking after us while my parents and older brother were gone during the day. As the day went by, my grandmother gave each of us one ptarmigan wing to eat. Near evening my mother and brother came back home. They brought back a lot of food. They brought two porcupine and a lot of fish. They also had killed some ptarmigan. I thought to myself, we will be all right now. My mother cooked some fish right away. In the evening my father came back with the otter he had gone after. Each day since we moved camp my father had killed an otter. That was the beginning for us to be all right and out of danger from starvation. From then on, fish were caught frequently. We kept on travelling around and soon we had the first spring thaw. We were not as bad off as we were and fish were caught more often from then on. After the spring thaw and the snow got hard again, we travelled to our spring break up camp site. 'After we get to the camp site, we will leave you there. I will go with our son to go and get the canoe,' he said to my mother. When we got to our camp site it was already very springlike. When we reached our camp site, we saw a bear going across the lake. My father went running after the bear. We made our camp. When the camp was finished, my father came back. He brought with him the bear's intestine. He had killed the bear. We feasted on the bear. It was the first big game that we killed since my grandfather's death. When my grandmother saw the bear, she thought of my grandfather. My grandmother started to cry because she missed her husband. That is where we made our camp. They left to go and get the canoe shortly after the feast. My mother caught a lot of fish. The spring was coming fast. My mother noticed that the ice had moved. A bridge had been made across the open water around the lake from the shore to the ice of the lake. My mother took out her fish lines. She made a lot of trips hauling her fish. She caught a lot of fish that day. The ice had started to dry up. 'We will not be hungry. The fish lines do not have to be in the water. We can live on the caught fish,' she said. Not long after that, we saw my father and brother coming back from their trip. The brought the canoe on a sledge. They brought some geese and ducks that they had killed all right. We ate. We waited for spring break up there. We were never hungry that spring for we caught fish often. But it was a different story for my uncle and his family. They had almost starved to death. Their bad luck with hunting had not changed since they left us as ours had. They only had broth to drink on very few occasions. Soon they were unable to move because of weakness from lack of food. During the first spring thaw and when the snow got hard again, they were already unable to move then. There was a man who was hunting around that area. The man was from the south of here. I do not know which town he was from. He had come for a visit here in Whapmagoostui but he never went back home because he liked it here. He had two sons and only one was married and the other one was still single. He had a lot of food because he had killed some caribou. He was travelling trying to get to his canoe. There was fresh fallen snow as they were travelling on that particular day. Their going was slow because they had heavy loads on their toboggans. His sons were going ahead. After a while, the sons saw something on the ice. When they reached the dark spot on the ice, they realized it was a fish line. They saw footprints on newly fallen snow. There was another fish line. They saw only two fish lines on the ice. From the footprints, the sons could tell that the person was very weak. They followed the tracks and saw them doubled back and onto the shore. They did not see any blood near the fish lines on the snow. They did not see any smoke from any dwelling. They realized what probably was happening to the people. They surmised that the people were bad off. The waited for their father to reach them so that he could see the signs of what they saw. When the old man came upon these signs, he right away realized what was happening to the people and that they were in a bad predicament. The old man went ashore by himself. He saw the dwelling standing there. When he got closer he saw some smoke, very weak smoke coming out of the dwelling. He did not see any firewood outside the dwelling. He saw footprints leading to a nearby tree and the person had snapped some branches and twigs from the tree. He supposed that the person got those branches to use as firewood. He called out. He heard someone inside the dwelling but could not recognize what the person was saying or who it was. The person inside the dwelling was already incoherent. He was the old man of the group. He said to his sons to get some water and to bring their toboggans ashore. He feared that they might not be able to save all the people and maybe some

*had died already. He did not see anyone of them sitting up and could not
tell how many were still alive. He just took up his axe to get some firewood
for the dwelling. He made a fire inside the dwelling and started to make
broth. The two youngest sons of the starving family did not recognize him
and were almost totally unconscious. These two boys he tended to first and
poured some broth into their mouths. He was able to revive them and
everyone was conscious later. He made the dwelling bigger and he moved
in with them. He brought in his food and gave food to the old man.*

The Whapmagoostui *Iyiyuu'ch*[6]

The Whapmagoostui *Iyiyuu'ch*, the people, talk about who they
are in terms of where their families hunted or continue to hunt
and in relation to other Cree communities to the south and east
of their region. They also distinguish between those who hunt
regularly and those who work in the village and only hunt on
weekends or during the goose-hunting season (Dick, 1991: per.
comm; see also Salisbury, 1986: 115, for a discussion of the polar-
ization between bureaucrats and hunters). However, the most
common distinction is the one made between 'northern' and
'southern' people, and is based primarily on where people were
born and where their families hunted and (in most cases) continue to hunt. Northerners are those who hunt, or whose parents
and grandparents hunted, at or near Richmond Gulf, Clearwater
Lake, Little Whale River, or Freshwater Seal Lake.

*The people who originally came from Richmond Gulf [before the post was
shut down] called the people from Great Whale River, 'southerners.' And
in turn, the people who hunted around the Great Whale River post called
the people who hunted near Richmond Gulf post 'northerners.' They give
each other these names.*

[Q: Are you a northerner or a southerner?]

*Of course, I am a northern person, that is where I was raised. That is
where I was raised to become what I am, I spent most of my time at Fresh
Water Seal Lake and further north. That is where my grandfather spent
most of his time. Way far, where 'the border' is [literal translation: the*

watershed, where rivers flow in the opposite direction], that is where he used to spend his time when he was still hunting. But I remember very clearly because I was already an adult. Way far north, at the barren land near Nastapoka River, that was where we spent our time for one year, all through the year because we didn't go to the trading post until the summer came. And that was how we always spent our time, like that, ever since I grew up. I spent my time at Fresh Water Seal Lake, also at Clearwater Lake, where the stream goes to the other side. That was also where my grandfathers spent their time.

Northerners are also those who may be from, or whose families travelled to, the Schefferville area and as far north as Kuujjuak on the shore of Ungava Bay. In the historical literature, northerners are described as Barrenlands caribou hunters; in this respect they are distinct from other Eastern Cree (Morantz, 1983; Francis and Morantz, 1983). Southerners, similar to other Eastern Cree, travelled as far south as Chisasibi and hunted inland and in denser boreal forest areas.

People in Whapmagoostui say that northerners and southerners have different traits, although examples of these are few and reflect biases held by the two groups rather than any particular traits per se. By and large the most important distinction made between the two groups relates to the large game they hunt. Southerners travel in denser forests and so have a longer history of trapping beaver. As well, for southerners the bear is the most symbolically significant animal (Tanner, 1979). Northerners historically hunted on the open tundra, where the caribou is by far the most predominant game. The caribou is a profoundly important animal for the Northern Cree, both as a resource and as a spirit presence (see Chapter 3).

One elder explained to me that even though he considered himself a southerner, there was no longer any great distinction between himself and other hunting families. Shifting migration patterns, he explained, meant that people could no longer be so readily categorized in this way. With the beaver and the caribou both so close to the Great Whale now, the northerners have taught the southerners about killing caribou and handling caribou skins, while the southerners have taught the northerners about beaver. 'So it seems,' he said, 'that right now they are all the same, what they do in the bush. They seem to make their living on the same things, like beaver and porcupine and caribou and fish and black bear – whenever they are lucky to get those things.'

Tacking between past and present, the people in Whapmagoostui today make different sorts of distinctions about who they are in relation to the land and to one another. The concepts *northerner* and *southerner* reverberate in every family's history, but today the dividing line between north and south relates not so much to *what* one hunts as to *where* one hunts. The village itself stands as the significant marker: those who head north of the Great Whale and up the Hudson Bay coast are northerners; those who cross to the south side of the Great Whale and continue south and inland to pursue their hunting are southerners.

People may also mention that they are members of a coastal community. While this implies, of course, that they live near water (as opposed to inland), the term actually derives from the relative degree of contact and not location per se. Of the nine modern Eastern Cree villages, five are deemed coastal and four, inland.[7] Today's villages and communities were first and foremost places where people gathered on a regular annual basis. As established meeting sites, they readily became settlement locations – places where trading posts were set up and where furs were exchanged for food, guns, ammunition, clothing, and other dry goods. The terms coastal people (*wiinipaakuu*; *wiinipaakw* translates to Hudson or James Bay, or to mean salt water) and inland people (*nuuhchimiiuiyiyiu*; *nuuhchimiihch* translates to the bush side, or inland) obviously locate the communities in the broadest geographic sense. However, the distinction between *wiinipaakuu* and *nuuhchimiiuiyiyiu* relates more to the accommodations that given Cree groups made regarding their trade, work, and hunting lifestyles. Those who congregated at coastal trading posts were likely to have more contact with non-natives and to work for the Hudson's Bay Company (HBC) – thus, the *wiinipaakuu* are those people who traded at the coastal posts through their hunting cycle and would have altered their annual travel routines to include staying and working at these posts for some length of time. The *nuuhchimiiuiyiyiu*, or inland dwellers, had relatively less contact and maintained a hunting lifestyle that did not include the same degree of accommodation (H. Bobbish-Atkinson, 1988: per. comm.; Morantz, 1983; Preston, 1981). Today the terms 'coastal' and 'inland' remain, but simply designate the obvious geographic and minor linguistic variations between the nine communities.

Richmond Gulf and the Little Whale and Great Whale rivers were common stopping points within the expansive boundaries of the northern Cree peoples' hunting territories. In other words, for as long as people can remember and long, long before any European presence in this region,[8] the mouth of the Great Whale was a regular summer meeting place for the northern Cree, who travelled up the Hudson Bay coast and as far as the Ungava Peninsula in search of caribou and other game. Small family hunting groups journeyed to the mouth of the Great Whale, where they reunited with parents and extended kin they had not seen since the previous summer. Marriages, 'walking out' ceremonies, and a variety of feasts and celebrations were held at this site. Young married couples saw their parents again, new grandchildren were seen for the first time, and news and stories were exchanged (Preston, 1975).

The Great Whale and Little Whale sites also provided an alternative source of food as well as highly valued fat. During the brief summer months the *Iyiyuu'ch* harvested beluga whale, which were once abundant in this region. The rendered whale fat was a highly valued food item that was carefully stored and transported, and used long after leaving the coast (cf. Walker, 1953).

The way the whale oil was eaten was with other kinds of game meat. It was good when some oil was boiled in with ptarmigan. It was best eaten with fish. The Iyiyuu'ch of the past were more apt to kill whales for its oil – as well as for food. As it was with everything else that the Iyiyuu killed for food, they handled the whale with great respect. When a whale would be killed, an old man was given the whale to oversee that the whale was shared and handled according to custom. An old man was made owner of the whale. He instructed that others be given part of the whale. He was the boss of the whale.

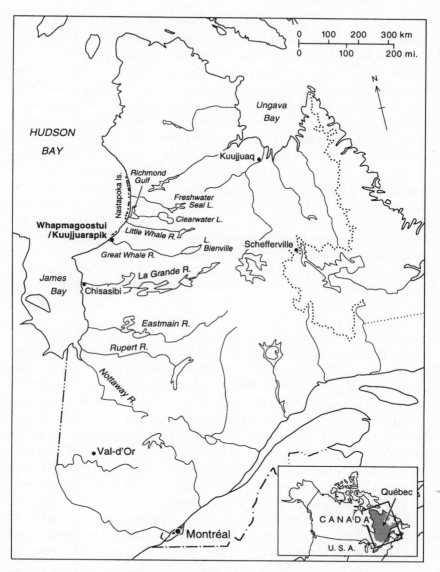

The northern Cree travelled in small family groups across the northwestern sector of modern-day Quebec, from Kuujjuaq on Ungava Bay coast to Schefferville,
the Little Whale River, Richmond Gulf, and the Great Whale River, and south to
Chisasibi. Following local practice, I am using the translated English names for
the region and its waterways.

The whale soon gained another boss: the resource was discovered by European entrepreneurs. During the early 1700s, the Great Whale and Little Whale rivers and Richmond Gulf – all of which drew Cree and Inuit during the summer months – were ideal locations for commerce between the native populations and European traders.[9] Both fur trading and mineral extraction were attempted at these sites, but neither succeeded as anticipated. Mineral deposits were never found in any quantity, and fur-bearing animals were not abundant enough in this taïga region. So while trade and some industry had already begun, it was not until whaling was established that the region became closely tied to the European economy. The brief excerpt that follows testifies to the magnitude of the harvest in this region. The European market for baleen and whale oil made this an especially lucrative resource. In particular, in the early nineteenth century, street lamps in England were lit with the rendered fat of beluga whales, many of which were harvested at the mouths of the Great Whale and Little Whale (Francis and Morantz, 1983; Marsh, 1988).

With an abundant supply of belugas at the Great Whale and Little Whale rivers, whaling was firmly established in the region by the mid-1700s. The Cree of this region, like the Inuit, were drawn more permanently to the coastal waters of first the Little Whale river and then the Great Whale to assist in the whaling industry. As skilled whalers, the northern Cree were easily incorporated into the harvesting, butchering, and preparation of the whales, and they provided the posts with much needed summer labour. Men were also hired to chop and haul wood, hunt for the manager's food, and perform other maintenance activities. Regular contact was clearly changing the seasonal hunting patterns of the northern Cree of this region. A minority chose to remain at the posts. Some stayed to work; others stayed because they were too sick to travel or because the fur-bearing animals were in decline. These were the first 'coastal' Cree.

The whaling operation lasted one hundred years, and was so extensive for so long that it virtually wiped out the beluga population (Balikci, 1959; Walker, 1953). With the advent of other forms

A Hudson Bay Company whaling expedition diary excerpt – 1814

July 1 – sailing from E.M. [Eastmain]

July 2 – anchored for the Night at Paint Hills [Wemindji]

July 15 – am at [Great] Whale R[iver].

July 22 – scaling north looking for better spot for the whale fishery

July 24 – am at LWR [Little Whale River] ...

Aug. 1 – set up boiling House (at GWR) – on the N. shore ...

Aug. 13 – ... oil taken on board the Schooner. 3 Tons of blubber from LWR, furs and deerskins, the latter retained for use at the house.

Hudson Bay Records 1814 (B.372/a/1)

---

of fuel at the end of the nineteenth century, the whaling industry began to decline. By then, the beluga were close to extinction. The few whales remaining were not anxious to be caught; one company manager at the Great Whale post complained that the whales were shying away from the river during the usual netting season and only entered the river after the nets had been lifted for the winter (Francis and Morantz, 1983). While the whale harvest dwindled, the post remained open, since the fur trade in the area continued to be reasonably profitable (Honigmann, 1962).

Profits increased as the Hudson's Bay Company, the dominant fur traders at this time in the North, began to offer incentives for successful trapping.[10] These inducements, combined with an increased reliance on ammunition and some purchased foods and goods – which were available only at the HBC post – encouraged more (but by no means all) of the northern hunting families to shift their base from the Barrenlands to the inland regions, where fur-bearing animals were more readily to be found. Speaking of the Inuit in particular (though the same can be said of the Cree, who also traded at the Great Whale post), Balikci remarks that 'it is easy to see at the beginning of this century, the main characteristics of the process of cultural contact: the technological changes that aided in the hunting of wild foods, the shifts in the rhythm of seasonal migrations, the increased dependence on the [Hudson's Bay] Company post (integration of Inuit into the modern economy), [and] the dominant status of the manager and the missionary in their interactions with the indigenous peoples' (1959: 73–4; my translation).

What is meant by this 'dominant status'? The missionaries and non-native post managers certainly believed they were superior to the native peoples of the North. This does not mean, however, that the Cree (or the Inuit) went along with this assumption. In particular, there is evidence that the Cree themselves chose how much they were prepared to accommodate non-native influences and commodities. For example, although some hunting families shifted themselves farther inland, most did not move themselves farther south toward the busier trading posts. The Hudson's Bay Company did not want to set up a permanent post at the summer whale fishery, and made the naïve assumption that as the fur trade grew, eventually the northern Cree would increase their trapping activity and move closer to a larger, permanent post farther south (Francis and Morantz, 1983; Balikci, 1961; Honigmann, 1962). But the Cree did not move as the European traders anticipated. As a result, posts were built, abandoned, and rebuilt within this northern region.

Also, integration into the modern market economy did not result in complete dependence on post supplies. The Cree maintained a considerable *inter*dependence with the HBC in this early period and traded only for particular goods that were of benefit to them. Caribou was still the most reliable food source for the northern Cree, as well as the one they preferred, and thus 'their independence [was] in the context of disinterest in those European goods other than ones deemed necessary for their survival' (Morantz, 1983: 64). The Cree traded primarily for small quantities of ammunition, metal tools, guns, twine, tobacco, flour, tea, and sugar (Morantz, 1983; see also Morantz, 1986; Francis and Morantz, 1983; Turner, 1894; Speck, 1915). Turner's ethnographic research, conduced at Fort Chimo (Kuujjuaq) in 1882–84, supports Morantz's findings: he found that the northern Cree hunting families who travelled to this post traded their furs for the gunshot, tea, flour, sugar, cloth, and string available there. On a practical basis, European traders never fully considered that there was a limit to the amount of trade goods or furs that could be hauled long distances on foot or by sled. Nor, for that matter, did they consider whether the Cree would want to embrace an economy based mainly on the accumulation of goods and/or wealth (Morantz, 1983).

Thus the northern Cree began to accommodate themselves to the fur trade. Some remained full-time caribou hunters; others went inland to trap; still others remained at and worked for the post (Morantz, 1983). The Whapmagoostui Cree had 'found a means of incorporating the European trade in a way acceptable to themselves and the HBC' (Morantz, 1983: 71). This pattern continued for decades. Most families continued to travel in their annual hunting cycles; the rest remained at the post either to assist with its operation or because they were too old or too sick to travel extensively (Walker, 1953).

Any history of the Canadian North would be incomplete without some reference to the Christian missionaries, who travelled to the most distant outposts in search of new converts. They first appeared in this region in the early 1800s, and are still very much alive in the stories of the Cree people. (Now, in the late 1990s, there are signs that some Cree are moving away from formal Christian doctrine, but that is part of the next vital chapter in the history of the Whapmagoostui people.)

While learning how to manoeuvre through the market system, the Cree were also exposed for the first time to organized religion. The early missionaries held the firm conviction that the native peoples were practising acts of the Devil, and this fuelled their resolve to convert the Cree to the ways of Christianity. As Edmund Peck summarized early on in his mission activities in the 'northern wilds' of the Hudson Bay region, 'Blessed be God that through my Saviour I am on the winning side' (1876, quoted in Petersen, 1974: 31). The missionaries were vigilant in their attempts to obliterate what they perceived as the barbaric ways of primitive peoples. In this endeavour, they left no room for indigenous practices; it was assumed that these practices were heathen and thus either dangerous or without significance or utility. Over

the years, and often after relentless effort, the missionaries succeeded in converting an entire people to at least some form of
Christian belief.

Christianity, and specifically Anglican church teachings,[11] had
a profound effect on the northern Cree. Yet it should also be
noted that often, despite the most stringent efforts of the missionaries, people acted in accordance with the Church while near the
post, but returned to the practices that were forbidden by the
missionaries – such as the shaking tent ceremony and other spiritual practices – while at their camps (Honigmann, 1962).[12]

In the eastern Hudson and James Bay region, the conversion to
Christianity was accomplished largely by two missionaries. Rever-
ends Edmund Peck and W.G. Walton exerted a profound moral
influence on the people of this region throughout the late nineteenth and early twentieth centuries (Barger, 1981: 673).[13] As
Leith and Leith note: 'Knowing every individual Indian ... dependent on Fort George and Whale River posts, and much of their
family history and having gained their confidence and respect,
Reverend Walton exercises a benevolent despotism over them
which extends beyond spiritual affairs. Anything he says "goes"'
(1912: 47).

*Even though they were only using arrows, that is how it was in the past.
But since people don't do what the people did in the past ... There was this
priest who came from far from here, his name was Mr Walton. He was the
one who stopped the people from what they were doing – like with the shaking tents.*

[Q: He was the one who told them?]

*Yes, he was the one who told them to stop. So, they stopped using the shak-
ing tent. He must have done the same with the people south of here, at all
the places he went to.*

[Q: But did he say why he stopped the people from using the shaking tents?]

*The reason why he stopped them is because he told them there is only one
thing we should think about as a Saviour, who we are living for each day
and everything that he made, and that is how it is written in the Bible. We*

should never think: What shall I live for? What shall I eat? How am I going to stay alive? We should never think that way. If someone thinks that way, it seems as if he has lost faith in Him. That is how the Bible is written, and that is how the people have been taught. That is the main reason why he stopped that. But, while they were still using those shaking tents, it seemed as if they had something else they could depend on ... Until the minister came all the way from England. He was sent because the other minister could not tell the native people like us – because they were scared to stop what the native people were doing. That was the reason he [Reverend Walton] was sent here because they were sure he would be the one to tell the people, he was the right one to do the job, to tell the Cree people to stop what they were doing in the past. That was what they did. It was the same with the Inuit. That is how the Inuit also changed, since the minister came to the town and all the other places, like Schefferville and all the other places because whenever the people noticed he would come to Great Whale, there were a lot of people who would come to see him, in winter, there were a lot of people who would come a long way just to see him, like the Inuit who would come by dog sled and in the summer he would travel by canoe, he would be taken to other places by canoe, with the large canoes.

Reverend Walton's words reverberate to this day in Whapmagoostui. Elders continue to tell stories of how Walton imposed his iron rule on the people and the community. Some now point to this indoctrination as the beginning of the end of traditional practices and communal social life among the northern Cree. Others see no contradiction between their Christian beliefs and their respective ways of life. People speak about how the pre-Contact ways were disrupted; yet those who are devout Christians do not believe that the imposition of Christianity damaged their traditional existence.

The Cold War and the Village

Over the past 300 years, a number of events and circumstances have affected the lives of the northern Cree and their relations with outsiders. The whaling and fur industries and the arrival of the missionaries are three obvious examples. In the past fifty years, these changes have been ever more swift and dramatic.

During the 1930s the region's animal populations – which are prone to natural fluctuations – began to decline as a result of overhunting. With neither food nor fur-bearing animals for exchange, the Cree entered a dismal period of hunger and poverty. Families remained on the land for the next two decades, living – and dying – in the only way they knew. As Honigmann found when he entered the region in the late 1940s, the Great Whale post was still serving only as a seasonal home for Cree (and Inuit) families. Fewer than 200 Cree, living in a separate camp near about the same number of Inuit, spent Christmas and the months of July and August at the Great Whale post (Honigmann, 1951, 1962; see also Twomey and Herrick, 1941). At this point the only permanent residents of the post were the Hudson's Bay Company manager, his wife, a store clerk, the Anglican missionary, and (occasionally) a federal radio operator.[14]

Rather than starve to death, more and more people began to move closer to the post, which was a source of at least some food and relief. This was a particularly difficult time for the Cree of the region, and life in the settlement was especially hard. Living in large family groups had never been uncommon; but when those same groups moved into inadequate settlement tents with little food or money, they grew hungry and weak, and tuberculosis, influenza, and other deadly infectious diseases spread rapidly. Extreme poverty, inadequate housing and sanitation, and rampant disease all became common at post settlements throughout northern Canada. Conditions, in other words, were deplorable, and they would likely have remained so for much longer had researchers not witnessed them and reported them to the federal government. In response, some health care and social assistance was extended to the northern native communities (T.K. Young, 1988b; Vivian et al., 1948; *Arctic Circular*, 1949; similar findings for Ojibwa: Moore et al., 1946).

So, I remember, too, the boat would come, people getting x-rays, I think there was a tent propped up. I remember when I was young 4, 5, 6 year old kid – dragged into a tent or some very bad place to get my x-ray taken, screaming and my mouth being pried open. So this was the first medical attention people were getting and then in the 50s when the DEW line was built, then there were permanent nurses and there was a doctor there, I guess to start things off, I don't know. First there were army nurses, I don't know, but there were about four of them, I think with the doctor to serve the base, but they were outside the fence, because it was fenced off. And so they looked after the people, started giving vaccinations then and I was 7 when I had my first vaccination and the doctors that were there, again, as always, as was expected, they were always gung-ho, saving people, or taking care of their medical needs and they went, and that first doctor who was here, I'm not sure how long, for 1 or 2 years, he would visit people's tents once a week even without ... even if people were not sick, he just came anyway to say, we are here, come on over, we have needles.

Not too long after these early federal medical assistance initiatives – and, significantly, with the end of the Second World War – the Canadian government instituted a nationwide welfare program. Given the terrible state in which the Whapmagoostui Cree found themselves, that postwar assistance was highly welcome. As people in Whapmagoostui explained to me, however, their parents and grandparents interpreted the welfare assistance in a different way than was intended. With only a limited understanding of postwar Canada, the Cree accepted the family assistance and welfare cheques as a proper form of exchange during these lean times. However, they thought the exchange was between the Hudson's Bay Company and the people directly, as it was the post manager who was in charge of dispensing the welfare cheques. More specifically, the post store was thought of as a local extension of the government – a logical conclusion, given the authority that the post managers tended to wield. Thus it was the store (as equivalent to the government) that was now providing the people with their subsistence. This made perfect sense and was viewed as a none-too-soon remuneration for all the furs the Hudson's Bay Company and the government had swindled out of the Cree in better times. After so many years of inequitable trade, and with a sense that the HBC and the government were one and the same, the Cree felt that the Hudson's Bay Company finally understood the wisdom of generalized reciprocity.[15]

Any short-term faith in fair exchange would be shattered in the years to come. As it turned out, the federal government was far more interested in the region than in the people who had lived and hunted here for thousands of years. In the summer of 1955, the armed forces arrived in Great Whale, and virtually overnight the settlement became a small armed forces base. It was the height of the Cold War and the military had been dispatched to the North to assert a presence and establish a string of Distant Early Warning (DEW) stations. Other, less remote, native communities in Canada had been aware of the Second World War and had actively participated in the war effort. Great Whale was still so isolated, however, that few of the people there knew about the war or the struggle between the superpowers that followed it. To this day, people recall their astonishment when they returned to the Great Whale site after wintering inland and found that buildings and high fences had been erected in their absence. Suddenly the region was connected to the rest of the world on a scale unseen since the decline of the whaling industry over a hundred years earlier. Suddenly, too, the local native populations had restrictions placed on where they could go. At this new army base, only military personnel were allowed past the barricades (see Balikci, 1959).

With the armed forces in Great Whale, a small northern 'town' emerged. Soon enough, a number of Inuit men and women made their way south to Great Whale, looking for construction and related jobs. The Cree also looked for these employment opportunities, but from about 1955 until the late 1980s, the village's Inuit population was greater than that of the Cree (c.f. Balikci, 1959). As the populations swelled, so did local animosities. Those who actually found employment discovered that along with the new-found incomes came unanticipated hierarchies and class structures. By 1957, Asen Balikci, working among the Inuit of Great Whale, found that '[l]es Esquimaux forment une classe de manoeuvres, de domestiques et de prostituées occupant la péripherie des grands établissement Eurocanadiens' ('the Eskimo form a class of labourers, domestic workers and prostitutes that occupy the periphery of the larger Eurocanadian establishment') (1959: 93, my translation). The Cree were treated with even less respect than the Inuit. Thus, despite increased employment opportunities and increased federal aid to those without jobs, an understandable hostility toward the newcomers persisted (Balikci, 1959).[16]

In 1958 the federal government decided to make Great Whale a permanent village, and for the first time established a health clinic, with one nurse in residence (Boulet and Gagnon, 1979). By 1960 there were 202 Cree, 375 Inuit, and 23 non-natives residing at the mouth of the Great Whale River during the summer months, each group with its own separate site (Johnson, 1962; Rogers, 1965). Johnson describes this geographic division: 'The village is neatly divided in two: to one side, the western, the tents and houses of the Eskimos; to the other, the eastern, the tents of the Indians. A stranger would not know where the Eskimo dwellings ended and the Indian dwellings began. And yet, there is no overlapping' (1962: 1).

The Cree and Inuit villages, always separate from each other, were now also segregated from the non-native community, which had arrived either to administer the two populations or to secure the northern borders of the free world:

North of the airstrip are ... the series of buildings which house the activities of the whites: the Northern Affairs complex, ... the apartments of the teachers in the school run by the Department of Northern Affairs, the school house itself, the nursing station, the large storage building which on Saturday nights and on special occasions is used as a community hall ... To the far east of this complex is the camp of the Department of Hydraulic Resources; to the west, the quarters of the Department of Transport, the Inn and the office of Wheeler Airlines and Nordair; and behind, fenced off from the rest of this little world, the self-contained life of the Mid-Canada [Distance Early Warning] Line base where well over one hundred white individuals lead their separate existence. (Johnson, 1962: 1)

The need for DEW line bases waned by the mid-1960s, and the radar base closed down completely by 1967.[17] That year the

federal and provincial governments jointly inherited full responsibility for maintaining the town and its people. With typical
bureaucratic aplomb, arising partly out of the federally desig-
nated division between Inuit and Indian, two entirely separate
federal agencies were set up to administer the Cree and the Inuit
of Great Whale (Barger and Earl, 1971). The Department of
Northern Affairs, which was responsible for the Inuit, maintained
an office in Great Whale. The Indian Affairs Bureau administered the Cree, but from a distance: their office was in Fort
George (now Chisasibi), roughly 200 kilometres south of Great
Whale.

As there was no local administration, the Cree did not have the
same access as the Inuit to government programs in housing, job
training, and education (Barger, 1977).[18] Inuit were hired over
Cree men partly as the result of local administration, and also
because it was perceived that the two groups differed in their
capacity to 'adapt' to town life (Barger and Earl, 1971). The prevailing logic was that the Inuit must be more adaptable to town
life since they could – and did – occupy the higher-paying skilled
jobs. This was hardly a fair assessment, given that the Inuit were
receiving better education and housing. The same opportunities
were simply not available to the Cree (Barger and Earl, 1971;
Wills, 1965). Wills found that even when the Cree requested
some of the financial benefits of the village and equal job opportunities, the Department of Indian Affairs would only finance the
production of handicrafts such as wood carvings. Barger and Earl
concluded that because of the preferential opportunities for the
Inuit, and because the Inuit perceived their traditional way of life
as harsh and unprofitable, they adapted more easily to town living
(1971: 30; Barger, 1981). In their summary of this situation,
Barger and Earl state that 'both our quantitative and qualitative
data indicate that the Eskimos have tended to move into the town
and adjust their life styles, in terms of activities and values, under
the new circumstances, whereas the Indians have tended to
remain more oriented towards their traditional way of life' (1971:
29–30).

Were the Inuit better off for having chosen town life? This was the accepted wisdom, which presumed a move toward (Western) acculturation and sedentarism (Walker, 1953; Barger, 1974, 1977). The Cree were extended little training, and few incentives to incorporate their hunting practices with wage labour, so it is not surprising that they were far less interested in accommodating themselves to non-native ways. More importantly, the Cree were assessing the impact this new 'town' would have on their way of life. They 'desired many of the benefits of the larger national society [but] were willing to participate in it only to the extent that they could *maintain their unique status and heritage, as Crees*' (emphasis added; Barger, 1977: 17; see also Salisbury, 1986). The Cree leaders were well aware of what their people might lose if they were subsumed within the village structure with its (restricted) employment opportunities (Barger, 1977). Once again, they accommodated themselves only partially to non-native ways, and continued to entertain a healthy suspicion of 'town' living. In the late 1960s the Cree of Whapmagoostui were still living in poor conditions, and animals were still in decline, and job opportunities were still limited, and yet they recognized exactly where they needed to focus their attention. The three main concerns of the community were spelled out by their leaders: self-government, land claims, and the preservation of their culture (Barger, 1980). The Whapmagoostui people could not have known just how vital each of these issues was to become to the entire Eastern James Bay Cree nation less than a decade later.

On 11 November 1975 – a date now celebrated in all eastern Cree communities – after a long and bitter struggle between the Cree and the government of Quebec, a historic agreement was reached that would profoundly change the lives of Quebec's Cree. This was the day that the James Bay and Northern Quebec Agreement (JBNQA) was signed between the Quebec Cree, the Inuit, and the provincial and federal governments. This agreement instituted the first native self-government in Canada. Yet it is what came *before* this agreement that would change forever the relationship between the Cree of northern Quebec and the rest of Canada.

Land, Self-Government, and Culture: The Fight Begins

It is worth repeating again and again that (then) Premier Robert Bourassa's 1971 plan to flood and dam the La Grande River in northeastern Quebec was arrived at without any consultation with the Cree people. 'James Bay I' was a plan to redirect and dam the La Grande River waterways in order to construct one of the world's largest hydro-electric projects. The Cree were caught entirely off guard, but quickly organized a new young leadership to fight the project. The long and arduous legal battles that followed resulted in the historic James Bay and Northern Quebec Agreement.[19] Although it was never anticipated at the outset of this fight, the agreement led to political, social, and economic changes in each and every one of the Cree communities. However, this was not a clear win or loss for either the Cree or the governments involved and the effects of the signing, both good and bad, resonate to this day.

Two stipulations in this agreement forever changed the relationship between the Eastern Cree and the governments that had 'administered' them for over one hundred years. First, the JBNQA, and the Northeastern Quebec Agreement that followed it, overrode the Indian Act of Canada for the Cree and Inuit of Quebec. Second, the Cree-Naskapi (of Quebec) Act that arose from the agreements established the legal basis for the first native self-government in Canada. While the Cree were finally free of the stranglehold of the Indian Act, this was still not a clear victory for them. Their new right to self-government is considered only a delegated right, not an inherent one (Cree-Naskapi Commission, 1986).[20] The Grand Council of the Cree of Quebec (GCCQ), organized to act as a unified voice for the Cree during the lengthy negotiation process, ultimately became the first regional government of the Eastern Cree of Quebec.[21]

Under the JBNQA, the James Bay Cree (and Inuit) of Quebec received benefits, payments, and land rights in exchange for title to 404,592 square miles (approx. 647 347 km²) of land. Also incorporated into the agreement is Cree control of wildlife resource management, as well as Cree and Inuit input into environmental impact assessments, a program of guaranteed income for hunting families, and guaranteed native economic and social development. Other fundamental benefits include administrative control over education, local justice, and local and regional governments.[22] As well, a Cree Regional Board of Health and Social Services (CRBHSS) has been created. The CRBHSS was established with a mandate to implement health and social service programs in Cree communities, and functions as a regional board under the Ministry of Health and Social Services of Quebec.[23] The JBNQA, in other words, offers the Cree (and Inuit) a means of subsistence, as well as community facilities that most southern Canadians take for granted (Salisbury, 1986).

The people of Whapmagoostui, although they were aware of and concerned about the effects of the hydro-electric project and the governments' activities, were relatively isolated from the political disputes surrounding the James Bay I project. As co-signatories to the agreement, however, they were involved in the negotiation process and benefited from the health, education, housing, and economic programs arising from the agreement.

In Great Whale the first and most visible effect of the JBNQA was that it formalized the division between the Cree and Inuit lands and people. According to the JBNQA, category 1A lands are those on which the indigenous populations have exclusive surface rights.[24] Category 1A lands have been used to build the new villages; also, uniquely in Great Whale, they have been used to create sharp boundaries between the Inuit and Cree communities. These formalized divisions have resulted in separate municipalities under autonomous Cree and Inuit jurisdiction. In the past, the two native groups were separated by federal versus provincial authority. In the present day, the Cree and Inuit function under entirely separate local governments, with autonomous schools, clinics, and municipal services (Boulet and Gagnon, 1979). For example, the Inuit village of Kuujjuarapik is run by an elected mayor and his council, while Whapmagoostui elects a chief and council. Of course, the Cree and Inuit have always spoken different mother tongues, hunted in different regions, and consumed different bush foods, and have tended to socialize within and live among their own kin groups. They even have separate church services. In other words, since the earliest encounters at this site there has rarely been much overlap of linguistic or cultural boundaries. Since 1975 and the creation of Category 1A lands, those boundaries have been even more sharply defined.[25] Suddenly, as well, unforeseen partitions have allocated lands and renewable resources according to an ethic of 'mine and yours' that runs throughout the agreement. In other words, an edict of ownership rather than usufructuary privilege has further divided the Inuit and the Cree (E. Masty, 1989, per. comm.). A case in point is the situation of a small convenience store owned by a Cree man. The front entrance of the store is on Inuit category 1A land, although the rest of the store sits on Cree land. The question arose at one time whether the store would have to contribute to the Inuit municipal tax on purchased goods. It does not – but the incident suggests the pervasiveness of the divisions between the communities arising from the stipulations of the JBNQA.[26]

Great Whale today thus consists of two municipalities: Kuujjua-rapik and Whapmagoostui. To complicate matters further, there are really *three* unofficial communities within the boundaries of these two municipalities: Inuit, Cree and non-native. There are, as well, two other names that similarly identify this tiny point of land on Hudson Bay: Great Whale River and Poste de la Baleine. The current total population is just over 600 Cree, around 300 Inuit, and 200 (mainly francophone) non-native people. Each of these three groups speaks a different primary language, yet they interact in a common second language: English.[27]

Except for the Anglican priest and his family and those few who have married into Cree or Inuit families, the non-natives in Great Whale live separately from the Cree and Inuit. The non-native teachers, clinic workers, government employees, Hydro workers, police, employment officer, court officers, postal employees, construction workers, and engineers all live near their offices. This entire section is north of, and referred to as being 'up the hill' from, the two native communities. There is minimal interaction between the native and non-native communities. Living in

Whapmagoostui, as I have done off and on for the last ten years, I have had only minimal interactions with non-native residents of Great Whale, and then only at the post office, airport, or general store.

Whapmagoostui has expanded radically (if not as quickly as was anticipated after the 1975 agreement), and the face of this one-time summer meeting place has been permanently altered. It is difficult to imagine that the move from the federally allocated slat-wood dwellings built in the 1950s into homes with running water and flush toilets began only in the early 1980s. Rents are set on a sliding scale, so that technically everyone in the community has equal access to housing. At the same time, the population is growing so quickly that, even with some new houses being built every summer, there are not enough homes for everyone. In some cases, families of three and even four generations must live in the same three or four bedroom house.[28]

The Cree village now includes a new band office, a school, a baseball field, an indoor hockey arena, a small grocery store, a radio station, a construction warehouse, a fire hall, and a machine shop. The other two stores, a church, a post office, an airport, an adult education facility, an employment office, a small hotel, a bar, and a snack bar are on Inuit land. So are all Inuit and non-native housing and all Inuit community facilities.[29]

Every year, roads of packed sand and crushed stone are extended, or new ones are made. The streets are used mainly by municipal services such as the school bus, the garbage truck, and snow removal equipment. Some individuals own cars, but most get around on snowmobiles in the wintertime and on all-terrain vehicles (ATVs) the rest of the year. For the snowmobiles and ATVs, the roads are merely a small part of the network of trails that weave through the village.

Land, Self-Government, and Culture II: The Fight Resumes

You must have heard what they have gone through, the ones who had a project on their land [the Chisasibi people]. Also we heard about other people who suffered from it and what kind of problems they went through and from our brothers. They were told how they suffered from it and we already know how hard it is going to be, we the elders know. Also we have to think about the young people who will be living in the future.

In 1989 the people of Whapmagoostui received word that the provincial government was once again looking north to expand its hydro-electric development. The JBNQA does leave some room for the development of northern resources – including the Great Whale River waterway – if the project's plans can pass strict environmental assessments. The original intention of the Quebec government had been to build the dams and power stations in the early 1980s. These plans were halted by a temporary surplus of hydro-electric power and a shift in government priorities. In 1989, with rising concerns about energy supplies, lowered water levels in the James Bay I reservoirs, and increasing costs of fossil fuel power, and with greater public opposition to nuclear and coal energy, the dormant James Bay II project was revived. According to the government of Quebec, the project would also provide a ready source of jobs in a depressed economy. The government anticipated that it would earn a substantial profit by selling the power to the Quebec aluminum industry and exporting it directly to the eastern American market.

The proposed James Bay II project[30] was massive. The plan was to divert three rivers north of the Great Whale River into an immense system of dams, dikes, and reservoirs; there would be three power stations at Lac Bienville, the source of the Great Whale River, and three more along the Great Whale itself, which would generate a maximum of 2890 megawatts of power.[31] To put it mildly, this project would have significantly altered the ecosystem of a vast area surrounding Whapmagoostui. It would have resulted in unknown changes to Hudson Bay, which would have affected the beluga whales, fish, and seals that migrate to and rely on these waters and their estuaries. Flooding, redirected water flows, and changes in water temperatures at turbine sites would have had unpredictable effects on the myriad bird and mammal species of the region. The Whapmagoostui people and their national leaders, the GCCQ, were fighting not just for the Great

Whale River but for other river systems on Cree land that were also slated for hydro development. The Great Whale project received the most media attention, as it was the first planned project, with work slated to begin by the end of the decade.

The Whapmagoostui *Iyiyuu'ch* care passionately about the river and the wildlife that depend on it and the vast lands surrounding it. After all, these lands were home to their parents and grand-parents, and their people had lived and died on them for as long as the Cree have existed. The massive project would never have made sense; thus opposition to it was virtually unanimous from the outset. In 1989 there was some talk by a minority of people that the jobs and projected road into Great Whale would outweigh any drawbacks of the project; also, there were a few otherwise unemployed people who worked for Hydro-Quebec's archaeologists as guides and camp hands. Ultimately, however, general consensus achieved precedence over personal advantage. The community voted to reject the project and to do what it could to halt the entire plan. Statements at meetings leading up to that vote argued against the project from a variety of perspec-tives. Pragmatic, legal and biblical arguments buttressed the Cree's position. At one community meeting in 1989, an elder spoke of the promise that God made to the people of the world, that this was a good Earth and that He would never flood it again. Another spoke of the potential for pollution and for changes to the local environment. Yet another reminded the audience of the scores of graves that would be flooded by these dams. As a result, the fish swimming above those dams could never be eaten.

The provincial Cree political organization had grown since the first James Bay conflict and had developed its own network of environmental experts and legal advisers. Also, a growing num-ber of young, university-educated Cree were taking active leader-ship roles. Compared to the obstacles the Cree had faced in their first confrontation with the Quebec government, this second campaign was eminently more successful in terms of the speed at which they were able to react. Clearly, the provincial government had not lived up to the promises written into the JBNQA. For that reason, it became increasingly difficult to enter into any new negotiations with either them or Hydro-Quebec (GCCQ, 1990; Copas, 1989). Before the end of 1989, and after the Whapmagoostui vote was taken, provincial Cree leaders decided to halt any further negotiations with either the provincial government or representatives of Hydro-Quebec. At the same time they were taking political and legal steps to terminate the project.

One local victory cannot be left out of this overview of the gruelling and frustrating conflict. In June 1991 at the Great Whale airport, a small army of Whapmagoostui citizens armed with little more than placards and their own voices succeeded in holding off an environmental review commission sent by Hydro-Quebec. ONLY BEAVERS CAN BUILD DAMS ON OUR LANDS read the signs that greeted these visitors. The Cree successfully blocked the hearings by not allowing these officials off the airport grounds or into the community (Hamilton, 1991). It made no sense, after all, to review a project that just could not happen.

Cree politicians were well aware of growing international concern for the environment, and knew they would find public support for their cause if they focused on the green argument. This was not cynical, but rather an astute and prudent assessment of the general political climate in 'southern' Quebec, Canada, and the United States. It is much easier to have the non-native public work at a level with which it can identify. The Cree concerns for the environment are not entirely consistent with those of non-native activists, who often deplore indigenous peoples' use of traps and the killing of the game and fowl. That being said, concern for the global environment is the rallying point of many disparate activist groups in the late 1980s and 1990s.

By February 1990, opposition to the Great Whale project had been organized under a coalition of environmentalists, trade unionists, religious leaders, and concerned native groups, who were asking for an independent study of future hydro-electric development in Quebec, as well as a moratorium on all planned projects (specifically, on the negotiation of contracts with the United States) (Communiqué de Presse, 15 February, 1990). Because of unresolvable differences between federal and provincial environmental agencies, the matter went to the Federal

Court of Canada, which ruled on 10 September 1991 that Quebec could not go ahead with the project without a review by, and subsequent approval from, the federal environmental agency (*Gazette*, 16 March 1991). By 1992 Quebec taxpayers realized how much the project would cost them. This, as well as support from Canadian and American environmental groups, added immeasurable support to the cause of the Cree. As well, investigations into 'secret' deals revealed that Hydro-Quebec was providing the industrial sector with energy at costs below those paid by household consumers; if nothing else, this kept the general public sceptical about the intentions of such a project as James Bay II. In 1991, frustrated by all these impediments, the Bourassa government announced a one-year moratorium on the entire project.

Lobbying by the Cree and their supporters, who by this time included environmentalist luminaries such as Bobby Kennedy Jr, led to the cancellation of important energy contracts in several northeastern American states in the early 1990s. Those cancellations, as well as the impediment of a very expensive yet flawed environmental review process and, significantly, a change in the Quebec provincial government in 1994, led to the quite sudden shelving of James Bay II in November 1994.[32]

Just as the battle for their land abated, another issue began to rise. The new Parti Québécois government, which had halted the hydro-electric project, was beginning once again to step up its sovereigntist agenda. Included in that agenda is the claim of sovereign title to all of Quebec, irrespective of signed treaties or agreements. Land and ethnocultural distinctiveness are, not surprisingly, the two most important issues being debated during this ongoing, fractious, and likely unresolvable dispute (Salée, 1995).

Where in all of this does 'health' fit? Health, say the people with whom I spoke, is the ability to negotiate the obstacles that threaten the survival of the Cree, be they environmental, social, political, or physiological. Understanding 'health' thus means understanding what it means to be Cree. I now turn to those meanings and connections.

Chapter 3

Miyupimaatisiiun: 'Being Alive Well'

They were miyupimaatisiiu because they lived in the Indian way, which was good for them. ... And the people said that's the reason why they were strong and healthy because they didn't use anything from the whiteman. ... That's why they were strong and miyupimaatisiiu, and that's what the elders knew. They were a kind of people, even if they didn't have anything much, they still would know what to do to keep well and strong in their lives. ... And that's how it was, before whiteman came.[1]

Sitting in the kitchen, or the living room, or sometimes in a *mii-chuap* (tipi dwelling), a small but conspicuous tape recorder at the ready on a table, and often with a cup of tea in front of us, the interviews would begin.[2] After a series of preliminary queries, I would turn to the one question that would invariably lead the men and women with whom I spoke into a familiar conversational pattern. It was the right and duty of the one who was speaking to tell all that he or she would on the subject. There would be no interruptions, except for a little clarification – a standard form of communication that privileges the speaker.

'*Chagwan miyupimaatisiiun?*' I would ask. 'What is "being alive well"?' Sometimes this one question would stimulate such a flow of stories that I was certain I would run out of tape. Other times, there would only be a few words. In all instances, however, people would reach deep into their own and their families' lives to tell me something of what it means to 'be alive well' – that is, to be healthy in the Cree sense of the term. Women and men talked about themselves and their families, telling their stories, histories, and legends; they regaled me with the successes and failures of life on the land and in the village. Evocations of the past were hardly what I had anticipated in a study of health. What possible connection could there be between 'health' and life on the land?

'Being alive well,' I finally came to understand, has everything to do with life on the land, and more broadly with 'being Cree.' In fact, the health of the northern Cree can only be fully understood within the context of the connections between land, health, and identity. Their discussions of *miyupimaatisiiun* moved discourses on health beyond the boundaries of the physical body by connecting physiological wellness to social and political well-being. Through stories and reminiscences, people speak directly to who they are, and through that they define what 'health' means to them. Linking past, present, and future, they narrate the path that connects the land to the people and to 'being alive well.'

Inevitably, that path also leads to the problems inherent in not being able to 'be alive well,' and to the intrinsic connections between this conceptualization of health and the politics of dissent. Everyone in Whapmagoostui must, of course, deal with the challenges of working or seeking work, raising and feeding one's family, growing old, caring for elderly parents, and simply making ends meet. Some must also contend with interpersonal violence, alcoholism, and sexual abuse. People did not shy away from discussing the agonizing traumas of hunger, sickness, and death that occurred in the past, or the contemporary hardships associated with village life. In this chapter I will elaborate the symbols and lived practices of *miyupimaatisiiun*, focusing specifically on its constituent elements: food, warmth, and physical ability. In the following chapter I will shift the emphasis to a discussion of the impediments to 'being alive well' and the links between *miyupimaatisiiun*, identity, and the politics of 'being Cree.'

Miyupimaatisiiun: 'Being Alive Well'

As I mentioned earlier, there is no word in Cree that translates into English as 'health.' The closest term is *miyupimaatisiiun*. *Miyu* means 'good' or 'well,' and *pimaatisiiun* means 'living' or 'alive.' Thus, in combination *miyupimaatisiiun* becomes 'he or she is alive well.' I intentionally use the more awkward translation 'being alive well' so that the term stands out in English as distinct from the more commonly used phrases 'living well' or 'well being.'[3]

The *Cree Lexicon: Eastern James Bay Dialects* (1987) translates *miyupimaatisiiu* as, 'He is in good health, he is recovering from illness.' I suggest that this translation is not accurate, except as an effort to translate a complex concept across cultures. As I will show in this chapter, the concept of *miyupimaatisiiun* goes beyond the simple statement that one is without infirmity.

Miyupimaatisiiun does connote, at a very basic level, the absence of disease, yet it is ultimately understood and described as something that goes well beyond the mere absence of disease. One is not only unhealthy if one has been sick; an individual can lose some of his 'well-being':

Twenty years ago, I was sick enough to be in the hospital for two years and I have lost a lot of my miyupimaatisiiun because of my illness. Even today, I see a doctor once in a while to see how my health is because of my sicknesses and because I am not very well.

Rather than simply 'he or she is healthy,' *miyupimaatisiiun* fundamentally implies that someone is 'alive well' or 'living well'; and this connotes a set of meanings that are contingent on Cree beliefs and practices.

The opposite of *miyupimaatisiiun* is not the negation of that word. *Nimiyupimaatisiiu* (the use of the prefix *ni* indicating a negation of the term) specifically denotes that a woman is out of her normal state of being. She is not unwell, she is pregnant. This is the only meaning suggested to me for *nimiyupimaatisiiun*. In Cree, the term that is more commonly used for being without illness is *nimintaakusin*, which is the negation of the term *nitaakusin*. *Nitaakusin* means 'I am not well, I am sick,' so *nimintaakusin* translates to 'I am not sick.'

The expression that may be used to indicate that one is not *miyupimaatisiiu* is *atuwaaitaakusiu*. This translates into English as 'she or he is lacking energy,' which is more a comment on that person's relative physical abilities. If a person is not looking the way she or he usually does and is sluggish or listless, or not carrying herself as usual, that person may be *atuwaaitaakusiu*. The term also implies that one might be weak from a lack of food.

My opinion about that and what I think it means is, where the Iyiyuu'ch are concerned in relation to the Iyiyuu way of life, ... all that the Iyiyuu was and had been before he [the Cree in general] used and integrated the whiteman's way of life into his own life, when he only used and lived his own way of life and used his own knowledge and lived accordingly and used his own knowledge to live the right way and to survive and did not abuse the knowledge that he had to live the right way in order to be well in all that he was, he was naashtaapwaa [very] miyupimaatisiiu. ... He only did all things that he knew that would only be to his well being and did only things that were morally right in his life and only did what would ensure his survival.

Warmth, Cree food, and strength form the essence of 'being alive well.' To be sure, there are other elements of *miyupimaatisiiun*; for example, for some Cree it includes devotion to the Christian doctrine. Cleanliness, too, is one of the fundamental principles of 'being alive well.' But Cree food, in particular, and warmth and strength, were pointed to again and again as the keys to 'being alive well.' 'Being alive well' is firmly tied to the ideals of living a Cree way of life – more specifically, a way of life imbued with robust connections to the physical and spiritual northern landscape. Indeed, there was a consistency in the way that 'being alive well' was presented to me that crossed gender, occupational, and to some extent age divisions. There is certainly a degree of diversity among individuals and households in what was and is done; what I recount here should not be taken as a static model of either concepts or practices. That being said, there was a congruity in how *miyupimaatisiiun* was described – a particular and consistent understanding and depiction of life lived on the land.[4]

Iyimiichim, Cree Food

What I use in my body that helps me to be miyupimaatisiiu, that is food that I eat and drink ... taking my age which is over fifty years old, I use the food we call Iyimiichim [from Iyiyuu = Cree and miichim = food] more than I do the food of the whiteman or food that is purchased from the store. That is what I like which is what I have seen when I was growing up. All that I ate was food that had been gotten off the land. Still at my age, what I prefer to eat is the food that the Iyiyuu kills to eat and every kind of food that is considered iyimiichim.

The things he knew from his own ideas, what he used and how he could feel good, the things he ate, what he ate, which would not make him sick, and it did him good, the way he prepared his food, and he had to kill for his food and he didn't have to eat anything which grows from the garden [implies things cultivated as opposed to wild], because the whiteman eats things from the garden. And the way Cree life was ... wildlife was the most important thing for them, and only what they made their living from.[5]

Iyimiichim are the food and food products procured from the land, water, and sky. They are the flesh, fat, and marrow of the animals, fish, and birds of the sub-Arctic. Cree food includes goose, duck, ptarmigan, grouse, porcupine, rabbit, otter, beaver, muskrat, caribou, bear, and, more recently in this region, moose.[6] Cree foods also include the fish that swim in the freshwater streams, lakes, and rivers throughout the inland forest.

For the most part, it is the Cree men who are responsible for procuring the meats that constitute Cree foods. The hunting of geese and ptarmigan and on up to larger game, such as caribou, bear, and moose, is done exclusively by men. Women may trap small game or fish, and they are familiar enough with guns – indeed, some women are quite handy with a .22 rifle. Even so, guns are the domain of men, and ultimately, shooting game is men's work.[7] When a larger animal such as a bear or caribou is killed, the animal is offered to an older man, often to one's father or grandfather.[8] This is done as a mark of respect to both the elder and the animal (see Tanner 1979). The elder will either decide how the meat is to be distributed, or pass that task back to the hunter. The large carcass is then butchered by the men and distributed within a single family or (in the case of a moose or a bear) among members of the wider community. Women may also distribute smaller game such as geese; and while some will be kept for future consumption – and especially for family and community feasts – a good portion of the surplus meat will be distributed through the kin network.[9]

Nowadays, food is usually distributed among a relatively small number of elders, siblings, and cousins. Hunted food is distributed first to the elders of the family, which may mean one's parents and grandparents and their brothers and sisters. Meat is also provided to members of one's family if, for example, others have been less successful in their hunting, or if no male household member is available to hunt. In the former case, there is a slight stigma attached to being the recipient of raw food, since this indicates a lack of success (see Tanner, 1979: 177). But when there is no male in the household, there is a decidedly restrained but appreciative anticipation of the meat.

The idea of redistribution is important to understanding the extent to which Cree hunters make their food available in the community. Redistribution maintains the strong bonds of reci-procity; it also provides bush food to those who do not or cannot live off the land (Driben, 1988; Feit 1991). Feit's discussion of the value of Cree food in Waswanipi is accurate too for Whapma-goostui:

In a society in which animals are sacred, and labour is highly valued and a source of respect, the bush food exchanges are highly valued. The gifting of bush food is both a sign of the value of those foods, and of the value of the social bonds which motivate the distribution. The fact that such exchange is less of material necessity today highlights its social dimensions. ... Gift exchange in foods thus flourishes, and reproduces the predominant value of bush over purchased foods, an evaluation of which cannot be explained simply by reference to biological need or by individual consumer preference. Rather food exchanges continue to express the primary commitment to sociality, and to recreating an active practice of mutual aid and responsibility in daily lives in which generosity is expected. (1991: 261)

Women, as part of their responsibility in maintaining the household, prepare and cook the meat and its accompaniments. The women also process the skins and furs. For larger game such as caribou and bear – and especially when that meat is eaten as part of a feast – the cooked meat is distributed by the elder male of the household, or in his absence by an elder woman.

The meat is prepared simply and with little seasoning other than salt, and is not eaten until properly and fully cooked, either by boiling, smoking, frying, or roasting. Usually the fish or meat is boiled or baked. When fish or meat is boiled, the rich, nutritious, and tasty broth (*muushkimii*) that results is also Cree food. The broth of most foods was once considered a proper remedy for a number of ailments, and an important first food if someone had not been eating for a long period of time because of starvation or sickness. In the past, I was told, fish broth was given to infants if the mother could not produce enough breast milk.

Animal blood is also a highly nutritious Cree food. For example, the blood and water that a goose has been boiled in is mixed with oatmeal to make a nourishing and hardy meal for young and old alike. Fat, too, was – and remains – a vital food in the Cree diet. A surplus of animal fat makes people feel prosperous and that the meal was both sumptuous and complete.

Once he had saved enough smoked fish, he could eat it with the oil. Once they got the oil, they would feel lucky to have it with them and they could eat it with anything because they hardly had enough meat to eat but once they got the oil, it made them feel that there was enough for everyone.

The food that was deemed to be the most important ... the caribou fat, was what the Iyiyuu regarded as the most important food and did not waste it in any way and [the fat] was handled with much care when prepared. For the [walking out] ceremony, the fat was taken out of storage [if it was available] for the feast and right on top of the fat, the ptarmigan beak was put and there it stood on top of the fat.[10] *When the child is taken out of the dwelling and when the child comes in again, it was said that whatever food that had been laid out was what he had killed. Then the feast began and everyone ate.*

In the past, people took the greatest care in rendering and then packaging the animal fat, ingeniously devising containers that could withstand the long and rough journey through the bush. For example, during the abundant days of summer whaling the rendered whale oil was collected and stored in a ballooned and dried whale stomach. The men then made

a box for the oil, because they thought it would be safer but they would put wet moss first on the bottom and on the sides before they put the oil bag in so it would cushion the bag, so it wouldn't break from the wood [box].

Despite the great care used to transport this ready supply of fat, whale oil, like whale meat, was never as highly valued as the meat or the rendered fat of land animals. *Pimihkaan*, or pemmican, a mixture of pulverized dried meat or marrow and animal fat, was a vital and easily transportable food source and remains part of the diet today. *Pimihkaan* is a very rich food and today is most often served as a special food at a feast. To this day, foods such as rendered bear fat are a favoured complement to meats, mainly because they taste good, but also because they are perceived as highly nutritious. Fat is an important and valued part of the Cree diet, although the heavy use of fat today is of growing concern for the Cree, and for Cree women in particular.

Cree food also includes the berries that women harvest in the late summer and early fall. Blueberries are still the favourite regional berry, but women may also collect bakeapple berries (*shikutaau*), the scarcer raspberries, and the quite abundant low-bush cranberries and blackberries. A popular summer meal is *shikumin*, which is a mixture of flaked, boiled fish and blueberries.

While berries are indigenous foods, flour, sugar, and tea are additions brought to the Cree by the early traders. These products are now considered staples and part of the traditional fare.

Bannock, in particular, is standard fare at many meals and is prepared routinely whether in the village or the bush. Bannock is a quick bread made from flour, water, baking powder, lard, and salt. It can be fried or baked, in the oven or over a fire. Often, the bannock dough is fried with fish roe or caribou meat; as a sweet treat, raisins can be added to it. For most people, tea is the beverage of choice. Indeed, it is rare to enter a home where there is not a large pot of tea on the stove; often it is made earlier in the day and left to cool to room temperature. Infusions of Labrador tea leaves or other locally picked plants are drunk, usually for medicinal purposes. Store-bought (Orange Pekoe) tea, although originally used mainly as a tonic, is now considered a staple – and traditional – beverage.

Iyimiichim and Cree Cosmology

With the few exceptions noted above, *iyimiichim* are primarily the animals that are trapped, hunted, or fished for food. More specifically, the animals are *iyimiichim* because they are part of a complex spiritual network involving the Cree people, animal spirits, and higher beings (Black, 1977, 1974; Feit, 1986; Tanner, 1979). In the Cree cosmology there is a rich and well articulated belief in spirit beings who can bring about, but are not wholly responsible for, successful or unsuccessful hunts. It was mainly the older Cree adults who were able to clearly explain to me the belief systems from which these principles derive, albeit often in connection with Christian doctrine. Among the younger members of the community there is a more ambiguous sense of respect for the land and its animals, which is often articulated not so much as a spiritual contiguity between the animals and the people, but rather as something that the elders teach the younger people.

In the course of daily life, the Cree articulate a deep respect for the bush animals. It is even the taken-for-granted norm against which youthful rebellious acts are measured. Those who impetuously shoot animals or birds are regarded as being wasteful and are made well aware by the community's elders that they have committed disrespectful acts. In discussions about hunting and wildlife, the word 'respect' is used regularly. Thus, while not everyone is as familiar as the elders with the animistic origins of the relationship between the Cree and the animals, people nevertheless articulate their relationship to the animals in terms of respect.

Proper respect must simultaneously be shown to the animals and to the animal spirits. The animal spirit beings are idealized conceptualizations of a particular animal, or group of animals such as land and water dwellers. The spirit exists in each of the animals yet does not die with that animal; it is a concept of a fluid force or vitality, and of a spirit that must recognize the hunter if that hunter is to be successful. That spirit, the *mischinaakw*, is not easily translated but can perhaps be described as the spirit of the animal that dwells simultaneously within all of its species and that also has the potential to live within a human being. Through this spirit the animal may become part of the (respectful and thus, good) hunter, dissolving any discernable boundary between person and the animal and between the natural and spirit worlds. Not all persons will have a *mischinaakw* inside of them; nor, for that matter, may they even know when they have a *mischinaakw* within; and some persons may have more than one. The evidence of having a *mischinaakw* lies in an individual's hunting success; the presence of a *mischinaakw* affords that individual a certain good fortune in killing that particular animal:

Sometimes, a person was well-known to have an easy time at catching fish. It was thought that the person who was good at catching fish knew the spirit called mischinaakw [in this case referring specifically to the spirit of water-dwellers] personally. I guess it is for that reason that the person had an easier time catching fish. I have heard my father say that some Iyiyuu were well known to be good at catching one particular kind of game, long ago. It was said that those who stood out as being good at catching that one kind of game, that they had the animal inside them but a very small one. The animal was always in their bodies. When this happens to a person that certain animal that he is good at killing is inside of him, then that is the reason the person is good at killing that kind of an animal.

Women are not excluded from this relationship to the animals and animal spirits, and their role is essential to the maintenance of the proper negotiation between the spirit world and the world of the Cree. The hunter is responsible for being observant and respectful when hunting; women must demonstrate the same respect at the camp. Women are responsible for maintaining a clean dwelling that is properly stocked with an ample supply of wood and water. Otherwise, animals may deem that dwelling unworthy of their presence and not want to enter it. Women are also responsible for the proper care and handling of the skins and meat of the animals. For example, Cree lore tells of the scorn shown by the 'Lady Spirit of the Caribou'[11] (*pihkutiskwaauu*) to those women who carelessly tanned caribou hides.

In the Cree animal taxonomy, animals are ranked according to their spiritual significance, their relative importance as food, and their degree of autonomy and self-sufficiency (Black, 1977). Since the caribou is the highest order of animal for the northern Cree, the Lady Spirit of the Caribou belongs to the highest order of spirits in the hierarchy of animal, human, and supernatural beings. The Montagnais animal taxonomy and language as elucidated by Bouchard and Mailhot (1972) provides further insight into how animals and humans are classified. The ranking is part of a broader classification of animals that includes three other elements. The hierarchy of power is associated with type of habitat, type of locomotion (four paws, flight, swim), and temporal-spacial distribution (seasonal migration). Each factor is dependent on each of the others; in combination, they provide a comprehensive picture of the relative position of each animal (Bouchard and Mailhot, 1972).

Above all animals and humans is a creator. Many today incorporate Christian doctrine with animistic belief and refer to this creator as God. God – or for others, the Creator – is the Supreme Being. God is the boss, as well as first leader in a descending order of assistants and lesser leaders (Feit, 1983). Melded with this is a sense of responsibility and self-sufficiency, and the knowledge that no one can act alone – even God has helpers. Thus, there must be a balanced co-operation among all parties within the hierarchy (cf. Black, 1977). Feit provides this illustration: 'In hunting, God is helped by the winds, with the "north wind" as the oldest, and the winds in turn are helped by the animal "masters," who are themselves the leaders of each kind of animal. And the old adults of each kind are the "leaders" of the young in a ranked chain of leadership and power' (1983: 16).

After the winds come the spirit beings of the high-ranking animals such as the bear and the caribou. Human beings fall somewhere between the animal spirits and the animals themselves. After humans come the animals. This ranking in the spirit world by and large complements the animals' relative size, strength, and value to the Cree. For the southern Cree, the bear is the most highly revered animal (Tanner 1979); in contrast, the Whapmagoostui Cree recognize the caribou as having the highest spiritual significance and nutritional value. Thus, the Lady Spirit of the Caribou plays a large role in Whapmagoostui Cree legends, because she exemplifies the highest level of wildlife. After the caribou (and the bear) are the smaller animals, birds, and fish.

The lowest animals are the ones considered both objectionable and inedible. Frogs, lizards, snakes, and all crawling or flying insects are classified as objectionable beings and rejected as food. Creatures considered unacceptable and inedible by the Cree are categorized under the general heading of *minituush*. While this term literally means 'maleficent spirits,' it implies something that is inedible for humans.[12]

The larger the animal a man kills, the greater his status. But animals are not simply killed – they are gifts that are *given* to a hunter who has acted in accordance with the principles of respect that guide his behaviour in the bush (Tanner, 1979; Feit, 1991). Once the animal chooses to give itself to the hunter, an unending cycle of reciprocity is established: 'To the animal which has given its life that humans may live, the hunter can only offer respect for its soul, proper use of its body, and sharing the gift of food with others. This incommensurability creates enduring obligation, which is expressed by participation in the wider network of gift giving, which eventually leads back to the rebirth of animals and renewed receipts of animal gifts; renewals which people say they experience in the continuing harvest of wildlife' (Feit, 1991: 237).

As befits a discussion of Cree beliefs, I turn to an elder to illustrate, through a story, the function of respect and obligation inherent in Cree cosmology.[13] The elder tells the story of a Cree person who lived a long time ago, before the Christian missionaries banned animistic beliefs and practices as heathen or worse. This was a time when hunters used to communicate regularly with animal spirits, often through an elaborate ceremony commonly referred to as the 'shaking tent.' The *mistaapaau* referred to in this story is the intermediary spirit who shakes the tent with its presence.[14]

The people would ... take care of what they had killed very well and handle it with respect so that they did not anger the spirits of the animals. If they handled the killed animals with respect, they would be successful in their hunts and the spirits of the animals would be happy to give food to them. That is the practice that the people kept always. They knew what the animals wanted, that they should be taken care of with respect and much care. The knowledge that they had about the wants of the animals is what they always tried to keep and practice. When they fail to keep these practices of care and respect of the killed animal, then they knew that the game was angered. Sometimes that was the reason why they did not kill food to eat. It is said that when someone really angered the animal that he depended on for food, the animal would leave that person [and hence, family] for good and starvation resulted.

This is a story of an Iyiyuu. There were two families living together. The Iyiyuu of this particular story was living with a family. The two hunters made a shaking tent. The mistaapaau told this to the one who made the shaking tent: that they will be killing some caribou. He was told that they would kill two big caribou and were given instructions about how to take care of these caribou. They had to be extra careful with these two caribou. The man was told that if he did not take care of the caribou well, it would be his last time killing anything. It was still the summer time. As they were paddling along, they saw two big caribou and they killed the two caribou. One of the men remembered what they were told and took extra care and handled the caribou with great respect and care. The other man remembered too, but he did not follow the instructions the mistaapaau had told

*them to follow when handling these caribou. Even though it was the mis-
taapaau who gave them the instructions, the mistaapaau was just telling
the wishes of the animal. In reality it was the animal [spirit] that gave
them the instructions on how to handle the animals [that were given to
them]. They killed the caribou ... To show the utmost respect for the animal, they did not eat it outside. They only ate the parts of the animal
inside a dwelling or some kind of a shelter. That is what the Iyiyuu did
first in the beginning. They did this to show how much they respected the
food and the animal.*

*One of the men and the one who was in charge of their affairs and was the
boss, was the one who did not follow what they were told to do. He started
making the fire and started cooking the caribou out in the open once they
had butchered the caribou. He gave some to the people he lived with, the
man and his own family. The other man told his wife, 'just wrap the food
because we can not eat it outside. We will eat it once we are inside our
dwelling.' After those two caribou were all eaten up, they were unable to
kill anything else to eat. The one who did not do what had been asked of
them said, 'make another shaking tent.' A shaking tent was made for him.
The mistaapaau went inside the shaking tent. They heard the mistaapaau
inside talking but the man could not understand what the mistaapaau
was saying to him. The people understood what was happening from other
people's experiences that they could not understand the mistaapaau
because he did not want to give them anything to eat [because they had
angered the animal spirits for one reason or another]. That was what was
happening. They could not make sense of what the mistaapaau was saying to them. The mistaapaau had also instructed them to take good care of
the caribou skin. Again, the man who was the boss did not heed the
instructions that had been given to them by the mistaapaau. The one who
was very careful had been given one caribou from the two that they had
killed. He had instructed his wife to take care of the skin well and to make
it very good and beautiful. When a shaking tent was built for the particular purpose of asking for caribou, the spirit that was spoken to was called
pihkutiskwaauu, 'the Lady Spirit of the Caribou.' That is the one that
was spoken to. That was the one who told whether caribou would be killed
or not and whether the caribou would be killed soon and when. I imagine
that it was a caribou that they were talking to directly ... The one who was*

not too careful was asked by the spirit of the caribou, 'I want to see for myself, to see how you took care of me.' The spirit said that, meaning it wanted to see how they had softened and tanned the caribou skin. The man could not show the spirit the caribou skin because it had not been tanned yet. The man who had been careful told his wife, 'Put the caribou skin that you softened and tanned inside the shaking tent.' His wife put the caribou skin inside the shaking tent. The caribou spirit was expressing its happiness and thankfulness about the caribou skin it was seeing, that spirit called pihkutiskwaauu. So, as it happened … he [the one who was careful] told the people he lived with that the end was near for them and that he would try his luck somewhere on a nearby lake. As soon as he had left the family he killed some caribou. As for the other family, I guess they perished because they could not survive themselves. The man and his family lived because he had done what he was told to do and he had pleased pihkutiskwaauu when he showed how well he had taken care of it. That is how and why he survived.

Disrespect in any of its various forms may have meant starvation and death. Even in the absence of shaking tents, the relationship between a hunter and the animals of the Subarctic is still founded on mutual respect. The culmination of the 'alliance' between the two is the moment at which the animal chooses to give itself to the hunter (Feit, 1986; Tanner, 1979). However, even the greatest respect does not always translate into success in hunting. People refer to the luck that a hunter may have, but that is a bit of a misnomer. A hunter's success is not so much a matter of chance as it is a negotiation of power between God, animal spirits, and humans. That 'luck' is also firmly grounded in a sense of one's fate in the world and of one's own abilities (Feit, 1991; Tanner, 1979). People today speak of the negotiation of luck (or perhaps destiny) and of a balance of success in hunting activities. There is more of a yielding to fate, along with a sense of what is expected behaviour – that is, showing the proper respect for the animals and a knowledge of the cyclical nature of wildlife. As Feit explains it, 'luck' is not random, but an indication of 'the ebb and flow of "power"' (1983: 18). Just as there are cycles in animal populations, so too are there cycles of hunting success.

The next story is about a man named Kakannapitat. Many versions of this tale are told in Whapmagoostui, some with greater detail, others with less; but all versions reveal the vital connection between humans, animals, and the animal spirits. As well, the story describes vividly many elements of the taken-for-granted hunting knowledge with which all children are raised. This is the story of The Man Who Never Killed Anything.

I'll tell you that Kakannapitat never killed anything. It was true that they knew he never killed anything, not even a bird, as he became a man. As his father grew old, they used to make fun of Kakannapitat. While he was walking, he was no different from any other man, but the only thing was that he never killed anything, not even a bird. Then he began to realize, 'I wonder why I ever became a man because I am very different from other men, which makes me look like a loser,' because he couldn't see or kill any animals like other men could. He took his bow and arrows and shot them just anywhere from where he stood until all his arrows were gone and he threw his bow away. Then he threw himself onto the ground and cried and he didn't remember what happened.[15] Then he woke up – there was someone – oh, I left something out, there was a Canada Jay who came by where he was lying, he saw that it was a man who was sleeping and he realized he didn't know this man, so he began to spread the news to his neighbours and he would say to them, 'I have found a man here, which means I never noticed him before – maybe one of you knows him.' It seemed as if all kinds of animals came to where he lay, which means all kinds of wildlife. And all of them told the Canada Jay that they had not noticed him before. The last one asked was the Lady Spirit of the Caribou, she was the last one to be told. And she told them, 'Of course, I did not know him, it was all of you who were supposed to notice him first,' she said to them. He woke up, and he noticed that someone was cleaning his hair. As he woke up, she [the Lady Spirit of the Caribou] said to him, 'No one noticed you before, that's why you had the kind of life you did, but things are going to be different from now on, since you've been discovered.' They told him which part of him they were going to be. The caribou, 'I will be in your chest because I will be a part of you.' And with the fish, 'I will be in the palm of your hand,' and he was told and everything else, they told him where they were going to stay, the animals which he was now going to hunt.[16] The

Lady Spirit of the Caribou said to him, 'I will take you for myself later, just because you hadn't been discovered yet because I would have known you before if they had noticed you,' she means the wildlife. 'The reason I am doing this is because the wildlife hadn't noticed you before – you will live forever once I take you. You will not die until the earth is destroyed,' she said to him. And the fish told him, 'I will be the first one you will search for, you will put the net in the water. As soon as you put the net in the water, the fish will come to it and the first fish you will catch, you will eat, and the second one you catch will be your father's, the third one will be your mother's. I'm only telling you what to do with just the three, the rest you can do with as you wish. A Canada Jay went wherever the man did, and when he got near his camp, he shot the bird and took it inside and the father was so happy to see his son carrying the Canada Jay. He told his wife to cook it right away and the parents ate it because it was his first kill, because the Canada Jay told him, 'you can do whatever you wish to do with me, if you want to kill me and take me inside, or not, right now, as you are heading home,' the Canada Jay said to him. And he was told which day he should search for each of the wildlife, all kinds of wildlife, one at a time, he should kill each just once in one day, that's what he was told. He also began to kill ptarmigan, that he was never able to before. Since the Canada Jay would go wherever he did, he killed one when he got near his miichuap [dwelling] and took the Jay in with him. The old man said, 'well, our son killed the Canada Jay,' he said to his wife, 'clean and cook it, I am going to eat it,' the old man said to his wife. And the man said to his mother, 'prepare the net, I am going to set it in the water.' They knew something was different because he had never said that before, and the mother prepared the net as she was told, it didn't take her long to prepare it. He took the net out as soon as it was finished and the elder ate the Jay. The elder ate the Canada Jay because he didn't want to waste it. He set his net right in front of their camp, he placed three floats on the net and the fish were caught as soon as he placed the net in the water. He continued with that, then he began to take out the fish that were caught in the net. The first one was a big one and the other one was also big, which was his father's so he was told, and the first one would be his and the third one his mother's. As he took the fish out of the net, more fish were caught, so he took the fish inside, and the elder was so happy and he said, 'this is the one I'm going to eat and this is my father's and this is your's,' he said to his mother. And the elder knew exactly why he was doing this, since he saw the change in his son. And the elder knew exactly what was happening. He had been told, 'you should finish everything all at once,' and he finished his own fish, and the old man finished his fish, but the wife could not finish, so the old man finished it for her – so the old man ate almost two fish. And he told his parents to take the net out because they wouldn't be able to eat all the fish, there were too many. They took the net out that evening before dark. And there were a lot of ptarmigan near their camp, and he shot them and put them inside. He went hunting and he didn't have to go far. He soon saw a caribou, a female caribou with her calves. He carried a small one home and the bear had told him, 'I will be the last one you will search for.' The beaver and the otter he killed just in front of his camp. So they had a lot of food because he killed all kinds of wildlife, also he killed a polar bear because he had been told that he should search for him. And he didn't have to go far, to search for the wildlife that he wanted to kill. And soon he wasn't able to move to another place because he had so much food which he could not move anywhere else. He knew that his son-in-law was near to where they were, the elder. They were told which lake they would be at, then he said to him, 'go and get your sister, tell her to come and help your mother clean the things that your mother is not able to because I don't think they have killed much food where they are,' the old man said. And he left to go to where his sister was, because he knew exactly where they were, and it was still daylight when he reached their camp, and the women who had always made fun of him said, 'We have a stranger in our camp and it is Kakannapitat. I wonder why he is dressed that way,' they said. Because they used to say that while the man is hunting, he used to decorate himself with the hide from the neck of the caribou, and that's how his mother had dressed him. And half of his arrows showed that they had been bloodied. And the women said, 'why does he dress like that? Because his father probably killed the caribou that was killed.' But he just ignored them when he heard what they said about him. Then his sister gave him some fish to eat and he said to his sister, 'the reason I came is because our father wants you to come to our camp because we found a lake which is very good for fishing and our mother cannot clean them all, because she is not able to clean them all, while we are able to catch some fish. And our father said that you probably are not having much luck with food.' His brother-in-law said, 'ok, we will move there.' It

was true that they weren't having much luck with food where they were.
And he told him, 'we will travel by canoe and then by foot when we get
near the camp. We can get the canoes later, we will come and get them
later,' he told him. And that night the man [son-in-law] said to his wife, 'I
think there is a change in my brother-in-law from the way that he was, I
guess he has just begun to hunt for some wildlife,' he said to his wife. And
he told the rest of the group that his father-in-law wanted him to come to
his camp. And they started their journey the first thing in the morning,
and he was in the same canoe with his brother-in-law. And he told them
when they reached the spot, 'this is where we will leave the canoe, we will
walk from here.' And wherever they were on the dry land, there seemed to
be a lot of ptarmigan around them. The other men wanted to kill them but
the ptarmigan were scared so it was hard to kill them for the other men,
but he wouldn't bother to kill the ptarmigan. When he reached where they
would leave the canoes and walk from, his sister told him – since there
were a lot of ptarmigan wherever they were, the men didn't give up trying
to kill the ptarmigan, the men from the group, and the ptarmigan seemed
to be so scared of them, and he would only walk with his sister and brother-
in-law the whole time – and his sister told him, 'hey, brother, why don't you
try to kill some ptarmigan?' his sister told him, and he said, 'ok, carry my
bag,' and as he went on they seemed to be everywhere he went. And it
didn't take him long to kill a lot. And they gathered them as he killed them
and the sister told the other women to take some for themselves because she
had already gathered a lot for herself and it was too heavy to carry them
all and they seemed to fight over them. Then he said to his sister that he
would stop killing them now – 'it seems that you cannot carry them all' –
and once they could see where the camp was, and he could see the pile of
caribou skins hung ready to be tanned and the teshipitaakin [cache made
of poles on high cut tree trunks to store meat above ground level], they
could see the cache and there were more than one. And they could tell that
the old man had a lot of food, by looking at his camp. And when they
reached the camp, the woman fed the people because she had prepared a
meal for them, especially her daughter. And she cooked a lot because she
knew how many there would be because she knew that they did not have
much food, and that's why she cooked a lot, so that everyone would have
enough to eat. So everyone was fed, then the elder said to the daughter, 'the
reason why your mother is not able to clean everything well is the reason

why I told you to come, the reason why I sent your brother to get you and all the things you see that have been killed, I, myself, have not killed anything, only your brother has – not even one fish have I killed, everything was killed by your brother. All the things you see here your brother killed it all. And I thought you could take whatever you can to clean for your own,' he said to his daughter. And he told her to extend their miichiwaahp so that she could live with her parents, the old man told his daughter. So they worked on their miichiwaahp to extend it because they wanted to live with them and while they were working to prepare their camp, the single women were discussing with each other, 'I'll be the one who will marry him.' And then one time, he said to his father that he doesn't want to be bothered by anyone, by which he meant the women, because they had made fun of him, 'if they don't do what I said, I won't be able to stay here with you,' he told him, 'if they don't do what I just said.' And the old man told his daughter to tell the women what he had been told, to warn the women, and tell them to stay away from him, that he doesn't want to be bothered at all. That's what he told his daughter to tell the women. Even though they were told, it didn't stop them, but I don't know how long it was, maybe it was until winter, it was in the winter, that was when he didn't return from hunting. He just didn't return from hunting while he was walking around his hunting ground. That's where he was picked up by the woman who told him that she was going to take him for herself, 'you are going to stay with me,' she told him. Then she told him to stay with his parents for a while, and he stayed with them for a while and again he didn't return from hunting, it was in the winter again. And that was the last time that he was seen. That's how it was told. [He left because the women were with him?] Yes, because the Lady Spirit of the Caribou said to him that he shouldn't be bothered by them because they used to make fun of him. 'So I will be the one you will be married to, and the reason why I'm doing this is because you were never described by the wildlife to me and if you were never described by the wildlife to me and if you belong to me, you will never die until the earth is destroyed,' that was what she told him.

Kakannapitat looked no different from any other man except that he could not kill any of the wildlife. He therefore could not be considered a man, no matter how old he was. Kakannapitat goes through a transformation when he loses consciousness of this world and awakens to find that he is from then on visible to the supernatural world of the animals. We learn how the animals must first become part of Kakannapitat, in other words – that he must be imbued with their *mischinaakw* before he can successfully hunt. Even the order in which they then give themselves to Kakannapitat is significant. Progressing from smallest to largest, from least to most significant, the animals give themselves to Kakannapitat in the order in which he would have hunted them through his youth, had he been a normal boy.

Implicit to those familiar with this tale is that the father knows through his own powers that his son has now been recognized by the spirits of the animals. Incorporated into the legend as well are the rules of respect and conservation – rules that are fundamental to Cree hunting practices. No food is wasted, and no animal is killed unnecessarily. Wastefulness is a sign of lack of respect and may be countered in the future by a change in the hunter's luck. The ethic of respect inherent to Cree hunting is tightly related to respect for the animals and the land, and to the humility that is part of an individual's relationship to these. Thus the elder in the story eats the 'weak' meat of the Canada Jay in order not to waste it, no matter how meagre the meal.

The ridicule that Kakannapitat had to withstand from the women divulges something else to the keen listener. How could someone wear the sign of having killed a caribou – the highest level of wildlife – they sneered at him, if he had never been known to kill anything before? To be a good hunter is to be a successful man – then and now – and when the women discover that he is indeed a very good hunter, they find him irresistibly attractive. Yet as the story ends, he chooses none of the women, fulfilling his promise to what seems to be a woman but turns out to be the Lady Spirit of the Caribou. In subsequent instalments of this tale, the relationship between humans and the spirit world is developed further as the man enters into the spirit world of the caribou. Ultimately, 'The Man Who Could Not Kill Anything' is an elaborate morality tale of relationships between humans and between human and animal spirits; it has a depth and richness that allows for new lessons to be learned with every retelling.

Part of how one shows respect to the Lady Spirit of the Caribou and to all animal life relates to how the men present themselves in the bush. Proper conduct in mediations with the animals is intrinsic to the concept of respect and to the hierarchy of power. It goes without saying that guns and vehicles must all be in as good working order as possible. Women play a central role in the men's preparations for the bush. For example, it is women's responsibility to properly make and decorate the outerwear. Foot-wear and mittens, as well as the gun cases, shell pouches, and hunting sacks, must all be well made and attractively adorned. As Tanner notes, 'It is the spirit of the moccasins and of the snow-shoes that lead the hunter to his prey, and prevents his legs get-ting tired, and thus those items are decorated to please these spirits' (1979: 92–3). To this day, women are also responsible for keeping the family's dwelling in good order and well supplied with water and chopped wood. If at all negligent in these duties – that is, if there is any sign of lack of respect – there is a risk that the animals will not see the value of giving themselves to the hunter and, hence, his family.

The Nutritional Value of *Iyimiichim*

As suggested in the story of Kakannapitat, the nutritional value of meat is connected to the significance of the animal powers or spirits. The larger and more powerful animals have a greater nutri-tional value and are thus viewed as stronger foods. Small birds have minimal nutritional value relative to the meat of either caribou or bear. Small birds are rarely eaten, so ranking begins with a more common food, the ptarmigan. Ptarmigan, a member of the pheas-ant family and fairly common in the region, is considered among the weakest forms of food and is ranked even below fish. Above fish are the larger migratory fowl such as ducks and Canada geese, then small game animals such as otter and porcupine, and on up to caribou, which 'is the strongest meat of all the wildlife.' Many of the older adults with whom I spoke discussed the relative strength of animal meats and cooking broth in relation to what one should eat or drink if one hasn't had food for a significant period of time.

Caribou meat was the strongest, as it was said in the past. If someone is almost starving to death, it was dangerous for them to eat caribou meat because it is too strong. It would kill him if he doesn't watch what he eats, it is better if he starts little by little, not to eat a large amount of food the first time because the meat is too strong – it would shock and kill him if the weak person eats it first, if he is dying from hunger. But they would know exactly what to do with a person, they would only give him a little, they would know how much to give that would be just right, they would start with a little amount, they would start with the broth. The stronger the person gets, the more the meat he can take.

Porcupine, and also its broth is very strong, it is very good to drink, it is good to drink when a person is weak from hunger ... With otter, it is very good to eat, it helps the strength, when a person is weak from hunger, it helps to get their strength back.

Bear or caribou would have been 'too strong' to consume after days of little or no food. Even the broth of these animals would be taken with caution. A preferable alternative to such strong foods was fish or fish broth.

The fat of the different animals has the same degree of 'potency' as their meat. Bear fat, for example, is considered very strong food and was used extensively in the past as a medicament as well. Animal fat, either alone or mixed with the inner bark of the tamarack, was used as a poultice on wounds or burns. Bear fat was described to me as an exceptionally potent healing agent – here, the animal's strength was reflected also in its curing abilities.

Beaver meat is anomalous in that it was considered, and still is considered by some, to be of less nutritional value than other animal meats.[17] One individual suggested that beaver meat was not perceived as increasing someone's strength because of the amount of work involved in killing a beaver in the winter. Another indicated that because the beaver is nocturnal in its habits, the meat and broth of the beaver is considered weak, irrespective of the amount that a person consumes.

Because the beaver doesn't do anything in the daylight, he only starts working at night. He works all night and rests during the daylight hours and that is what he is and that is why his broth is weak for regaining one's strength, even if he has a lot of fat on him. Even if they would get full from the beaver meat, it would still not do them much good for their strength. Even if they would get food from the beaver, they would still get weak. The beaver and the ptarmigan are considered the weakest foods or broth for someone who needs to regain his strength.

Finally, there are foods that are given preferentially to either men or women. Some people spoke of the very explicit symbolic meanings attached to certain parts of animals; others simply told me that men or women just don't eat those foods (cf. Tanner, 1979). These divisions, hierarchies, and preferences apply only to bush animals. Purchased meats such as turkey, chicken, pork, and beef hold none of these meanings or values.

Fish, fowl, and bush animals are butchered in ways that pay heed to these gender distinctions. Sometimes certain parts of an animal are given to either men or women in order to ensure future luck with hunting. For example, various parts of the goose are considered better for men (or women) to eat. The goose's head should be given to young hunters so that they may have good kills in the future; women eat the feet so that the geese will be drawn down from the sky. The wings and gizzards of geese are also considered women's food, although no reason why was suggested to me.

The heads of most animals and fish are considered men's food; so are the tails of porcupine, otter, and beaver (the content of which is pure fat). The jaw, nose, eyes, and tongue of the caribou are considered delicacies and at the same time men's food. One woman suggested that 'mostly the nicer parts' are reserved for the men, although women can and will eat these foods if they are offered (cf. Tanner, 1979). Tanner further explains that the head of an animal connotes honour and so is always given to male hunters. Fish heads are thus an example of a food that is given preferentially to an older man or woman. At Whapmagoostui, fish heads are considered a delicacy, but this choicest part of the fish may be offered to an eldest daughter or son.

Women who are premenopausal and girls who are not yet of child-bearing age are not permitted to consume the meat of any fetal animal or any part of the reproductive organs of female animals. A woman is not allowed to eat these organ meats in part because if she does, her children will not be able to come out of her own womb. In the same vein, women are advised against eating the 'balloon' of the sucker fish, since it resembles the amniotic sac. If eaten by the mother, the baby will not be able to 'break out of its bag.' Postmenopausal women can eat all of the previously proscribed foods, but they may choose not to.

A caribou fetus may be left untouched (Tanner, 1979) or it may be eaten, but strict rules apply to its care and handling. The fetal caribou is handled with great respect and is the first thing prepared by the women if a pregnant female caribou has been killed. At spring goose camp in a year when caribou were more plentiful than geese, I was watching two young hunters butchering a caribou when they discovered a fetus inside. The family matriarch called out from the *iyiyukamikw* to have me bring the fetus directly into the dwelling. It was handled quickly, efficiently, and with proper respect, all the while the elder woman explaining that this had to be the case lest anything happen to her daughters' young or yet to be born children. Leaving other work aside, one of the daughters carefully cleaned, dried, and skinned the animal. The soft hide would be used as a decoration or for a child's clothing, but not for footwear or mittens or for any other ordinary use. The meat was cooked and eaten first by the elder woman – since there was no elder male at this camp – and then by the younger adult men. In the past, the hide of any fetal animal would have been kept as a talisman and used as part of an appeal to the Lady Spirit of the Caribou for a successful hunt, as a means of indicating how proper care and respect had been shown to the animal.

Inedible foods include not only those which are symbolically disvalued (*minituush*) by their ranking in the hierarchy, but also those which are considered symbolically dirty. Animals that eat garbage are, quite simply, dirty animals. For example, seagulls are not eaten because people do not want to consume their own waste, which they see the gulls feeding on at the dumps just out-side town. The following two comments highlight known and feared (symbolically) dirty foods.

Whenever the Iyiyuu sees an animal that is usually food for the Iyiyuu feeding at a garbage dump, the Iyiyuu know right away that the animal is no longer fit for us to eat. Even if the Iyiyuu sees the just the animals tracks or only sees the animal walking near garbage, he right away thinks that the animal cannot be eaten any more.

The bear will catch the [fish] sickness [i.e., mercury poisoning], too. Also, the bear will not be healthy to eat because it will eat food from the garbage dumps [when the hydro projects are built]. The caribou will be sick, too because of the damage to the land because when the explosives are used and the drilling, the dust from these things will go up in the air and deposit on a large area over the land. The caribou eats its food which is the caribou moss and other plants, therefore the caribou will be sick, too, because its food will be damaged, too. That is how the caribou will be affected. It is very likely that the humans will be affected too because of eat-ing the caribou and other animals who eat the caribou will be sick, too. That is where the reasons will come from for [the Iyiyuu'ch] not being miyupimaatisiiun.

Obvious in these statements is the connection between what the animals eat and the land and water upon which they depend. These interviews were conducted in 1989, when the threat of the hydro-electric project was very much on people's minds. Thus, the two elder men connected dirty, polluted, and altered land to dirty, polluted, and altered animals and ultimately to dirty, pol-luted, and 'unhealthy' humans. This same theme was repeated in other interviews when people explained that Cree food is pure because it derives from pure land. Only animals that eat clean food can be clean and pure (cf. Lacasse, 1982).

The other thing that I have found out is that it helps one to be on the land because it is always clean and pure out on the land. Wherever the person is, it is always clean and pure. That is what helps the person for his well being.

In the past everything was so pure, that is why people were so well. And there was nothing in the water which could make people sick, there was nothing from the air which would affect the lakes because there was nothing disturbing the land ... They were hunting on clean land, that is why they [were] so miyupimaatisiiun. Especially the children, they [were] miyupimaatisiiun because everything was clean/pure at that time, the water, the land.

The mercury that now permeates the fish and the cadmium found in caribou and moose organ meats are understood by the Cree to be directly related to whiteman's activities.[18] Once again, Joseph Masty Sr's words echo the sentiments of the people of Whapmagoostui: 'If the land is not healthy then how can we be?'

Starvation

Starvation and hardship were recounted so often in the interviews that these things merit particular attention. The meaning of the term starvation is contested in the literature; so is the degree to which people actually went without food or specifically without meat (Black-Rogers, 1983). Writing over a century ago of the Cree who travelled as far as the Ungava Peninsula, Turner remarked, 'Although their food consists of reindeer, ptarmigan, fish and other game, the deer is their main reliance, and when without it, however great the abundance of other food, [the northern Cree] consider themselves starving' (1894: 276). Seventy years later, while working in Great Whale, Wills found that 'the Montagnais-Naskapi speak of the past as a time when the Indians were very poor. Even though game was more plentiful than it is today, they remember the hardships of trapping and many cases of starvation, and recall that white men present at the time did not help Indians who starved' (1965: 30).

I presume the suffering and the hunger to have occurred inasmuch as it is part of what is remembered and retold. Stories of starvation were recounted as stories of the cyclical availability of foods or changes in the hunter's 'luck' with the animals (cf. Tanner, 1979). People discussed with me how they or their ancestors overcame periods of little or no food, and how entire families had such 'poor luck' that they all eventually succumbed to starvation.

The time I remember, I was old enough to hunt ptarmigan [approximately seven years old, sixty years ago], I was lucky only sometimes in my hunting. There were a lot of people leaving from here [Great Whale] to go north to Clearwater Lake, a lot of families were there. Those are the people who died of hunger … [There were] five families. One family, for sure, everyone in the family died of hunger. Of the five families, only one daughter got married and is still alive. She is my next door neighbour. When there was hunger, it was the men who were first affected because they had to hunt, then the children, and especially if there was a mother breastfeeding a baby because of the baby sucking milk from the mother. Seventeen people died of hunger.

When no large game was available, fish were relied on. Not being able to harvest any fish was a sign of desperation.

If someone doesn't have enough food to eat all the time, if they were short of food – fish was always good for everyone, it would help them keep their strength.

As mentioned earlier, lichen was resorted to in times of utter despair. The black, scaly, crustose lichen that grows on rock surfaces in the Subarctic region was collected, boiled with water, and eaten as a thin porridge when there was no other food available. It was neither palatable nor nutritious.

The prevailing consensus is that there were dire periods of starvation during which no meat or fish could be found and entire families succumbed to hunger and cold. At the root of *miyupimaatisiiun*, at the very core of 'being alive well,' is the ability to 'be' in the most literal sense. To be able to withstand hardship is the true test of *miyupimaatisiiun*. To be 'be alive well' is to be able to withstand the hardship of little or no food while others perish. This is the greatest test of endurance and strength – the characteristics that both define and result from *miyupimaatisiiun*.

The Effects of Cold on *Miyupimaatisiiun*

Exposure to cold weather or cold water not only makes one sick but can also decrease one's ability to 'be alive well.' Staving off the intense cold that characterizes the long Arctic winter is fundamental to 'being alive well.' And once again, there are many stories that serve simultaneously as histories and as cautionary tales in detailing the consequences of negligence. The pragmatics of survival are integral to everyday life even today, whether the setting is the bush or a modern dwelling.

One is always warned about water and the cold. One is taught how to look after one's self during the cold weather. The other things people are cautioned is to be careful when they are using axes and guns. These are the most important things that they have to be very careful about. These things were already in the knowledge of the Iyiyuu of the past and handed down through the generations.

Precautions against the cold are taken by people of all ages but especially by those with infants and young children. Infants are not exposed to the outside elements at all until near their first birthday, and whether indoors or out they are securely wrapped and bundled in a *waaspisuuyaan*.[19] Originally a 'moss bag,'[20] nowadays a *waaspisuuyaan* is a soft fabric bunting bag. Wide strips of caribou skin trim the two front panels, in which holes are punched for thinner hide strips, which are looped to secure the infant inside the bag. Inside the *waaspisuuyaan*, the baby is dressed, her head covered, and she is wrapped cosily in a flannel blanket. The baby's feet are wrapped in infant-style moccasins, and in the winter, the mother may wrap a small piece of rabbit fur around her baby's feet for added warmth. In the past, the *waaspisuuyaan* was fixed onto a cradle board; nowadays, when taken outside, babies are secured on their mothers' backs inside a large woollen blanket, which is wrapped and knotted around the mother's midriff. In colder weather the infant is then completely enveloped in another large blanket before being taken out of doors. To not take such care of one's children is to risk their lives and unnecessarily raise the ire of family and friends, who would equate such inattention with cruelty. The following story illustrates the dire consequences of inattention.

It was because she did not tend to her right away when she cried while they were travelling [the child was being carried in the toboggan]. It was said that the woman was like the person who was not very kind and loving. She did not seem to show much loving care to her children. Her child was crying while travelling and she was carrying the child in her toboggan. She did not listen when the child told her, 'Mother, I am cold.' I guess the child had been moving about in the toboggan. I suppose the mother had not put mitts on the child [even though she was wrapped in blankets while in the toboggan]. What is done when people have things to do that is to dress the child warmly even though it is wrapped up and kept warm while being transported on the toboggan. The child is carried on the toboggan and mitts are still put on the child's hands. When the child manages to expose her/his hands out from the wrappers, [then] his/her hands are kept warm. It is presumed that is what happened to child [exposing her hands out of the wrappings]. It was not known if she had put mittens on the child. She did not care to check when the child said, 'Mother, I am cold.' I can not tell exactly what happened because I was still very young when that happened. But I did see the child as a woman. On one hand all her fingers down to the knuckles were gone and just the thumb was there. On her other hand, the whole hand was gone. I do not know exactly what happened to her hand ... I remember her while she was still alive. She lived despite her ordeal. The old woman was there when this happened ... I do not know what they used on her. I suppose they just used tamarack, I presume. I could imagine that they also used seal fat, I really can not say truly, if they were near the post. The seal fat was used at times and helped the Iyiyuu, just like I told you about the beaver fat, when these fats are used raw. It could be that they used seal fat, whatever fat it was, to oil the tamarack to put on the wound ... If she had not kept on walking when the child said, 'I am cold,' if she had not done that, if she had turned around to check and believe the child when she said, 'Mother, I am cold,' her child would not have gone through this kind of ordeal. The child would not have had frozen hands because she would have fixed the wrappings and tied her more securely on the toboggan and warned her not to expose her hands to the cold. She should have done these things. It must have been easier for the child to put her hands out because she had not secured her well in the toboggan. She was known to be like that, too, one who does not keep her children's clothing well and secure. She did not seem to be able to work well as she should. She did not seem to care much for her children. She did not work much.

Hard work was expected of both men and women in the bush – survival simply depended on it. To survive, however, sometimes meant that additional safeguards above and beyond the physical warmth and protection found in the *waaspisuuyaan* were needed. In the past, a small necklace made of netting was placed around the baby's neck to 'trap' the cold before it could enter the baby's body, to spiritually shield the baby from the effects of the cold (Flannery, 1962).

They would make a small necklace with thread and put it around the baby's neck and they would say, 'This little net is to keep away the cold so that the baby would not catch the cold, to protect her from catching the cold.' It helped a baby, but it's just that not everyone had the power/exper-tise [chi kischitaau] to make a net for the baby, so that when a person made the net, it would protect the baby from the cold. I knew ———'s mother ... had the power, making the net for the infant to protect it from the cold. Also, my grandmother who raised me [had that magical/spiri-tual ability] ... [They used] the kind of thread they make a net [ahapii] with ... They can see sometimes, when the white faded, if you could see a different colour, not white any more, that means it's protecting – the cold is stuck on the ahapii. It's the same thing as if you are catching a fish with your net, it's the same thing that you would say, that the net is protecting the baby from the cold. When the net loses its white colour, they would wash it and then put it back again after it is dried.

Some still make and use this protective neckwear for newborns, but its use has been discouraged over the last few years by individ-uals concerned about the safety of placing a string around a baby's neck.

Learning to protect oneself from the cold begins at an early age and continues right on through adulthood. Adults always dress in enough layers to protect themselves from the cold, especially when travelling any distance. Travel to and from goose camp is done either by Skidoo, or all-terrain vehicle (ATV), or canoe, and men and women don the appropriate outerwear for the trip. Head, hands, and especially feet are shielded from the risk of cold or inclement weather.

There is no question that one should always wear the appropriate protective gear – although, as an important aside, I must note that the definition of a strong Cree individual is one who can readily withstand the cold, even with minimal outerwear. Many stories of great men of the past are stories of those who were able to survive the harshest conditions with only minimal clothing. These stories detail the fortitude and strength of the Cree. It goes without saying that few if any non-Cree could survive in similar circumstances. Today there is a general distinction made between the Cree, who are hardy enough to withstand the sub-zero weather, and the non-Cree, who must take extra precautions when outside in the winter. I know this both from stories told to me and from first-hand experience. I was a subject of concern every time I ventured out of the village: 'Be sure your feet are warm!' 'Where is your hat?' 'Does she have enough on?' 'Will she be cold?' This vital concern did not, however, always translate into appropriate action on my part. On our travelling party's arrival at spring goose camp in late April 1989, word of my inappropriate footgear reached the family matriarch before I did. As soon as our Skidoo pulled up to the cluster of tents, I heard a familiar voice calling me: I was to come directly to her tent, remove my boots, and sit with my feet to the fire until the chill was gone. Of course, I did so, and when my feet finally thawed, I assured the elder – and myself – that I would never again be so foolhardy.

Concern for oneself in general, but especially for one's feet, is crucial to survival in the Subarctic. Having cold *and* wet feet is especially distressing and warrants a stop on even the shortest outing. The functional importance of walking and of one's feet is underscored by the spiritual importance of the lower limbs.

Although not articulated today as explicitly part of an animistic belief system, great attention is paid to how one dresses for travel in the bush. One's feet, in particular, are treated with special importance, and footwear such as moccasins and snowshoes is always colourfully decorated (Tanner, 1979).

If someone gets cold or chilled, it is unquestionably a cause for concern. Allowing cold to enter one's body, whether by accident or by not dressing properly, threatens the loss of bodily strength. Once cold enters into the body, it continues to reside there until driven out. For this reason, people take great care not to get cold and act quickly if someone becomes cold. People who retain cold in the body or who are repeatedly exposed to undue cold eventually become sick. Prolonged exposure to cold has a cumulative effect that leads to lung, joint, leg, and other problems over the years.

Like the ones who have leg problems, the ones who have leg problems, it's because they got cold, they got cold because they spent a lot of time outside, especially when they had to spend the night outside during a cold winter, and once they got cold, it would stay inside and build up inside them and that's what would make them sick. That's what happened ever since I started to have the pain and it stayed there. Once it's there, it will always be there. Also, it's the same for women, the women have the same problem – when they get sick, it's from the cold. They also have leg problems, as if they can hardly use their legs, that's what the doctor said. If they haven't been treated right away to sweat out the cold, by using the rocks, that would help sweat out the cold. That's the only way, to sweat it out. Once it's sweated out, even when it is deep down, but if it isn't sweated out, if someone got cold, especially if he got wet and cold, and sometimes it would go to his lungs and that's what he knew.

Women must be especially cautious of exposure to the cold since it can adversely affect blood and particularly, menstrual activity. It can even interfere with childbirth. Today, girls and women are instructed to keep their feet warm at all times. This prevents unnecessary menstrual pains and ensures fewer physiological problems in old age.

For the girl, it is dangerous for her to get cold because of what the woman has [menstruation]. That is why the female child is taught to watch that she does not get wet or watch that she does not get too cold for long. If a girl gets cold before her first period, that is why she will not be well. I heard long ago that a girl got cold before her first period and the blood came out through her mouth instead of the other way. That is why it is dangerous for a girl to be cold while having her period ... I also heard that it went to her head and her mind was affected because she had been cold [too often].

The usual treatment for someone who has gotten cold is to replace the cold with heat. Routine heat treatments in the past included using a steam tent/sweat lodge (*mitutisaan*), or surrounding the afflicted body part with hot stones and covering it all with a cloth.[21] Today, people consider a hot water bottle a somewhat adequate replacement for the localized dry heat treatments of the past.

One thing that the steam tent [mitutisaan] is used for is when a person feels chilly all the time and feels shaky inside as if being cold. That is what I have seen a person using the mitutisaan for that purpose because they have been cold and [the cold] had been retained in the person. That is why the mitutisaan is used to bring out the person's cold water that is inside of him.

The Iyiyuu gives heat treatments to someone who is known to be cold through before the cold goes to the lungs. Once the cold enters the body, if it does not come out to the surface of the body [in the form of sweat] it travels straight to the lungs. When the water that is supposed to come out does not, that is what happens. The whiteman says that it is not good for someone to sweat when someone is very sick. But the Iyiyuu has a different idea about this. When a person has been cold, it is advised that the person have heat treatments whenever possible before he gets too sick from his being cold thoroughly recently ... When a person sweats, they feel good and relaxed after their sweat session. The water and the cold come out of the person's body. Sometimes, the person is known to have the condition of having been cold because their sweat is cold to the touch. It is said that the person's state of having been cold is coming out. The Iyiyuu administers heat treat-

ments to the person who has the condition of being cold. When fate deems the person to live a long life then the heat treatments work.

In this statement we again encounter a sense of resignation to a higher order – the logical fate of the individual who must be self-sufficient but who ultimately has no final control over his or her destiny. This same yielding to fate – though hardly with resignation – was discussed in relation to all treatments as well as in relation to hunting success and, more generally, in all vicissitudes of life. It was always accepted that if there was no improvement after three treatments, the person was not meant to get well.

Being able to withstand the cold is a clear sign that one is 'alive well.' In much the same way, if one is not 'alive well,' that person may become chilled, which in and of itself increases the likelihood of a range of illnesses. Many people said that people in the past were obviously stronger and better able to withstand the elements than the people of today; they were very *miyupimaatisiiu.*

Those people [in the past] must have been tough, the ones who could stand the cold water ... not to get sick from that. But if any of these people right now would do like they did in the past, I'm sure they would get sick right away. I'm sure they would feel sick right away if they got wet from the water – that is how dangerous the water is, if someone gets cold from the water, it would affect the person right away.

Physical Ability

Physical ability, in terms of strength and endurance, was one of the principal elements discussed when people spoke to me about *miyupimaatisiiun.* Specifically, to 'be alive well' one must have the physical endurance to withstand the cold and to hunt and prepare food. Thus the qualities that are most closely associated with *miyupimaatisiiun* have not changed over time – only the ability of individuals to actually 'be alive well' has. As far back as I can remember, said one elder woman,

when the Iyiyuu says someone is miyupimaatisiiun they mean the person

*who never seems to be tired out even though they have not stopped working
all day long. Someone who can lift heavy things but is not tired or never
known to be feeling sick because they are tired from working and doing
things all day long.*

One must be strong enough to carry out the activities necessary to survive in the bush. The more physically active one is, the
stronger one will be. At the same time, the only way to acquire
that strength is to eat Cree food, and the only way to get Cree
food is by hunting.

In the past, industry and tenacity were signs that a person was
truly 'alive well' and also that he or she had the ability to help
others be 'alive well.' Thus each member of the group was linked
to the others through reciprocal obligations.

*When a person did not let up in pursuing his work, which some Iyiyuu
excelled at doing this, it really showed in their lives because then they had
good and prosperous lives. He alone made it possible to live the well and
prosperous life because of his industriousness and hard work and he also
made it possible for others to [be] miyupimaatisiiu. The reason why it was
possible – that is what I heard tell and not from my own experience do I
know this – is that it was his enthusiasm and industriousness towards his
work that gave him the miyupimaatisiiun and assurance of his own survival. An Iyiyuu with that kind of attitude towards his work did not know
what it meant to be lazy at all nor did he like to be lazy in any way. It was
this kind of attitude to his work that also gave him the knowledge of how
to do well in doing and pursuing his work for survival. He did not like to
be lazy or to be doing nothing.*

*But there were times that the things they liked were not within reach.
Whenever the Iyiyuu'ch were at the post just a while, they were very anxious to be getting back to the kind of life they were living which was being
in the inland and living off the land. The kind of life they were living and
liked was on the land and the knowledge they had for this kind of living is
what they taught their children as soon as they were able to understand.
One of the things that was good that the Iyiyuu'ch taught their children
was to wake and get up very early in mornings and never to sleep into the*

*day too much. The habit of the Iyiyuu'ch to get up before the sun was up
was a habit that was practised all their lives. That was what they did all
the time. They never slept late into the morning. They hardly ever stopped
doing anything for a while. They always kept themselves busy with the
work that needed to be done. At my age, which is over fifty, what I like is
what I have seen while I was growing up as a young child.*

*I knew and I heard that there were many people who wouldn't easily get
tired even if they work so hard and carry heavy loads many miles, but still
they wouldn't get tired easily, that's how the people were a long time ago. It
was just because they would eat the wild animals that they would kill and
it was before they would eat any other different kind of things ... That's
how strong the people were in the past. That's how the people were when
they made their living only by hunting.*

*That's the main thing, that people got strong and miyupimaatisiiu
because they moved around all the time. They would work hard everyday because they knew they were miyupimaatisiiu enough to do hard
work.*

That one has been out hunting indicates that one has the physical strength needed to survive in the bush. Physical strength is
also evidence of an experienced hunter and of a woman who has
the skills required to prepare the meat and hides. Also, there are
integral links between physical ability, *miyupimaatisiiun*, and bush
activities.[22]

*The people were miyupimaatisiiun because they were always travelling
and were used to the life they had even if they travel for miles and miles,
they would probably rest on Sunday but start on Monday, but they were
used to the life they had. I knew and I heard that there were many people
who would not easily get tired even if they work so hard and carry heavy
loads many miles but still they wouldn't get tired easily, that is how the
people were a long time ago. It was just because they would eat the wild
animals that they would kill and it was before they would eat any other
different kinds of things. That is what my grandfather told me. That is
how the people were when they made their living only by hunting.*

The Iyiyuu of the past age never depended on anything to carry them from place to place. They depended only on themselves to get to a place even if the place they wished to go to is very far. They made their own transportation with their body energy and nothing else carried them wherever they wanted to go. They carried their own belongings in winter and in the summer. Since the existence of the posts, the Iyiyuu went to those posts, even though they were far from wherever they might be, taking their pelts, if they needed anything from the posts, and they were fast at it, too, it is said. Once they were on this kind of expedition, they were very far from where they started from in one day because they walked with great speed. They only ate when they were camped for the night. That was the only time they drank, too. While they were walking during the day, they did not even stop to drink, much less stop to eat but only when they were camped for the night. That is what the Iyiyuu of the past did. They did everything with great speed, too. That shows that the Iyiyuu of the past were miyupimaatisiiu.

So that is what happens when a person is slowed down by hunger – mostly it was hunger that slowed people down when they were miyupimaatisiiu. But the people never knew when to stop, they would always overwork themselves. … Because mostly if they don't eat as much as they should that slowed them down, so they were supposed to always have enough food to eat to keep them going because they had such a hard life, to make their living.

Summary

If the hydro project cannot be stopped, considering the damage and the loss that will be done to the land, this will also speed up the loss of the Iyiyuu way of life, therefore, the Iyiyuu will not be miyupimaatisiiu, in essence, the factors that enabled the Iyiyuu to be miyupimaatisiiu will be destroyed and lost for them.

Protection from the cold, physical activity, and eating Cree food are the main factors associated with 'being alive well.' Closely bound to this concept are respect for bush animals, devotion to Christian doctrine, cleanliness both in the house and in camp, and the proper handling of food. Furthermore, there are particular foods and abilities that contribute to well-being but that are meaningful only in the context of Cree knowledge and lives. In other words, concepts of well-being are bound to 'traditional' Cree practices and cannot be dissociated from Cree ideology. *Miyupimaatisiiun,* say the adults that I interviewed, is synonymous with the Cree way of life, and is inseparable from being able to hunt, pursue traditional activities, live well in the bush, eat the right foods, keep warm, and provide for oneself and others. *Miyupimaatisiiun* evokes a past that was characterized by living on the land, for the most part unencumbered by whiteman's interferences, foods, and illnesses. The past envisioned in these stories does not exclude any of the harsh or demanding conditions that were inseparable from that lifestyle. Many stories focus on the difficulties of survival; often they are stories of death – sometimes of entire families – by accident, disease, or starvation. In this vein, the enduring and abundant Cree ethnomedical knowledge reflects a close understanding of hunger, starvation, accidents, and infections, as well as treatments for these. As well, in the oral and documented records, there is a high incidence of infant mortality and of deaths of mothers during or just after childbirth (T.K. Young, 1988a, b). Life was indeed hard – but outside of the influences of whiteman.[23]

Discernible throughout this chapter is a certain self-consciousness in explaining what is 'really Cree' and, thus, how one can 'be alive well.' As Feit explains for the case of bush food, 'The value of bush foods may also reflect the fact that bush food production has become a symbol for distinctive Indian identities, Indian skills and knowledge, and Indian rights, in the midst of increasing contact with local and national Euro-Canadian society' (1991: 261).

I agree with Feit and suggest that food production and consumption are two of the fundamental elements that distinguish Cree identity. Cree well-being is connected not only to eating Cree food but also to the sense that Cree identity is currently in jeopardy. The links between 'being alive well' and being Cree, and differences between Cree and non-Cree, are central to my discussion of the political nature of health. 'Being alive well' is central to what it means to be Cree, and can only be achieved through separation from all that is perceived to be non-Cree. Clearly, Cree individuals feel better – feel healthier – when they are in the bush, practising a Cree way of life and eating Cree foods (cf. Tanner, 1979). This way of life is exactly what is at stake in the battles against a steady stream of Euro-Canadian encroachments. The Cree ideals of the 'balanced participation with the world' (Feit, 1986: 180) have been tested repeatedly over the years; and in the face of that, the ability to 'be alive well' is being steadily lost by young and old alike.

Chapter 4

The Politics of *Miyupimaatisiiun*

Much as the people with whom I spoke could not escape the links between *miyupimaatisiiun* and the history of living on the land, I cannot escape the connections between identity and personal, social, and political well-being. At one level, *miyupimaatisiiun* means that a person is able to pursue those activities associated with hunting and bush living: eating the right foods, keeping warm, and maintaining the viability of the group through sharing with those in need. These activities are in turn a constituent part of a larger cosmological order in which animals and humans exist alongside their spiritual counterparts. This is a fundamentally simple message of a history of survival in a northern hunting population. Yet that message also speaks to a profoundly different perspective on health. 'Being alive well' is never just individuated biological fitness or wellness. For the Whapmagoostui people, 'being alive well' is always contextualized within a configuration of individual and community beliefs and practices. Those beliefs and practices are in turn forever located within the vicissitudes of histories as they are remembered, lived, or even just aspired to. Health is thus coupled with identity, and as such is confined neither to the boundaries of individual bodies nor to biostatistical normalcy.

In this analysis of Cree conceptualizations of health, what is of paramount importance is how the people whom I interviewed chose to explain what 'being alive well' means to them. Debates around authenticity and representation are meaningless to the people of Whapmagoostui. Far more meaningful to them is how, despite the many gains they have made through the JBNQA, their lives and livelihoods have been dramatically altered in the past few decades. Thus it is hardly surprising that they turn to their past in order to articulate their personal and collective sense of well-being.

This relationship between *miyupimaatisiiun*, history, and identity stems as much from the very real sense that a hunting lifestyle is preferable for the Cree as it does from the realization that recent changes are having an increasingly harmful effect on the community. Recall that there is clear evidence of a historical relationship between Cree and non-Cree that can best be described as a form of relative accommodation. As I laid out in Chapter 2, the Cree did accommodate, if not fully incorporate, the goods and services flowing into the North. However, the more recent history of relations has not been one of accommodation. As federal and then provincial interests imposed themselves more and more deeply into the North, there was less incentive to accommodate to the needs or the will of the State. At the same time, there has been increasing reflection on the past, and in particular on the time (imagined or not) when living outside the constraints of those impositions meant living a healthier life. It seems, then, that the greatest obstacle to *miyupimaatisiiun* is not disease, but that which impedes 'living well.' The greatest barrier to 'being alive well' is, quite simply, said the people, 'whiteman.'

Waamistikushiiu – 'Whiteman'

Waamistikushiiu – 'whiteman' – is raised again and again as the greatest impediment to Cree well-being.[1] *Waamistikushiiu* refers to 'white man/person,' to people from far away, or to English-speaking people. While there are other terms for francophones and for people of other nationalities, the word that is used most often, and that generally connotes any non-native outsider, is *waamistikushiiu*. This word not necessarily derogatory, but neither is it a term of endearment. *Waamistikushiiu* is that homogeneous 'other' – an entity, if not an individual per se, that stands in opposition to all that is considered Cree.

There is an interesting character, still regularly spoken about, who epitomizes the potential malevolence of 'whiteman.' *Pwaatich* (pl.; *pwaat*, sing.) is the term the Cree use to refer to the non-native men who used to travel 'eight to a canoe.' The original *pwaatich* were the map makers and prospectors who travelled on and around the Great Whale River during the nineteenth century and who gained a reputation for persistently threatening the safety of the Cree people. *Pwaatich* harmed people directly by injuring or killing them, or indirectly by stealing their food (see also C. Scott, 1984, 1989a). In a more recent incarnation, *pwaatich* were linked to the military personnel who were stationed at Great Whale in the 1950s (cf. C. Scott, 1984). People described *pwaatich* to me as white men who lurk in the thicket, awaiting their prey – young children and especially young girls. To this day, the children of Whapmagoostui are warned from an early age – and only half in jest – to beware of *pwaatich*.[2] For example, they are told to be quiet and especially not to speak English when walking in the bush, lest they lure the *pwaatich* to them. Stories recounted to me use *pwaat* interchangeably with the word for 'whiteman,' although *pwaat*, in particular, always implies someone who should at the very least be avoided. *Pwaatich* has become an imagined spectre, one who exists just beyond the boundaries of the Cree world and who epitomizes 'whiteman's' uncharitable and unkind behaviour (cf. C. Scott, 1989a).

The mythic malevolence of *pwaatich* is matched only by the pervasive inequalities the people see being imposed in the various spheres of daily life at Whapmagoostui. Even though this is a self-governed Cree village, a surprising number of disparities exist. From the rigid medical clinic routines to the structured church services to the recently defined boundaries that divide the landscape into municipalities and circumscribed hunting zones, the Cree now find their lives cross-hatched with constraints and conditions. For example, nurses who are not native and who don't speak Cree are often perceived as unsympathetic to Cree medical complaints and to the routines of the Cree community. Why, one individual asked, can we not get an Aspirin at night (when the clinic is closed) or before heading off to hunting camp? Because there is no pharmacy in the village, the people depend heavily on the clinic for all their medical needs, and they feel that the routines being imposed by the clinic staff limit access to the only health facility available to the community.

Waamistikushiiu is also directly associated with diseases previously unknown to the Cree. The infectious diseases of the last century, as well as the more recent scourges – diabetes, asthma, heart disease, cancer, and AIDS – are all widely understood as whiteman's diseases.[3]

In Whapmagoostui, even one's choice of food underscores the divisions between Cree and non-Cree. 'Do you want spaghetti or *iyimiichim* [Cree food]?' asks a father of his young daughter, imbuing the choice with a meaning that extends far beyond simple nutritional value. In the grocery store, the rows on rows of tinned foods, the all-too-often wilted and blemished fruits and vegetables, the sweets, and the processed foods – all exorbitantly priced and all whiteman's food – are further reminders of whiteman's material impositions. Whiteman's foods, when eaten in quantity, directly affect the health and strength of the Cree person. Whiteman's food has the potential to imbue those Cree who consume it with whiteman's (negative) characteristics. In other words, these foods are symbolically polluting and weakening (cf. Douglas, 1966; Meehan, 1982). As a corollary to this, going without indigenous foods for any length of time is potentially harmful to the well-being of Cree people.

The things that children ate in the past, that was what made them strong and miyupimaatisiiu – because they ate only wildlife food, because they only killed what they needed for food. With the whiteman's food, sometimes it doesn't do a person well in his system if he eats just whiteman's food for a long time. But if he eats half wildlife food and half whiteman's food, that would do him all right.

Of course, people purchase, eat, and enjoy many of the foods found at the grocery stores in Great Whale. In fact, canned and prepared foods have become something of a routine necessity, for they are handy to transport and eat in the bush and (more often) when a quick meal is called for in the village. That being said, these foods are always regarded as whiteman's foods, and a distinction is always made between purchased foods and *iyimiichim.*

Bush food is still the food of choice; it is the food that was meant for the Cree, I was told. Many adults remarked resignedly that eventually the children would probably be all right since their bodies would get used to the variety of foods they eat today. Yet many still feel that people today, and especially the young people, are somehow weaker and less able to perform a range of Cree activities because they are not eating enough of the proper foods, and more specifically because they are eating too much whiteman's food.[4]

Confusing for some are the apparent contradictions between the categories of whiteman's foods and the relative availability of those foods on the store shelves. Local public health campaigns suggest that some foods are better for you than others. Why is it, then, that the most 'unhealthy'/bad foods to be found in such abundance at the grocery store? For some Cree, the confusion stems from the practice of ranking foods according to their nutritional value. If it is a food item and it is being sold, then why shouldn't one be able to eat it, even if it is *waamistikushiiumiichim* and thus not nearly as strong as Cree foods? This dilemma stems in part from how Christian doctrine has been interpreted. One of the fundamental teachings of the church, say many of the elders, is that God has put everything on the Earth for the good of all humans. It follows that not to consume any particular food item makes no sense. On the surface, this way of thinking is illogical, since this religious doctrine was a non-native imposition to begin with. Over the generations, however, and with the melding of Christian doctrine and Cree beliefs, the question has come to revolve less around the origin of belief or practice and more around the incongruity between a food's availability and its value. Even so-called 'whiteman's tools,' such as guns, skidoos, and central heating, are now accepted because they are not only helpful but part of a far greater order – an order that presumes the beneficence of God. Then how is it possible, elders ask, that some foods (or goods) can be bad for you if they are just more of God's creations? They know, of course, that store-bought food is not Cree food and therefore not good for the old people and likely damaging to the constitutions of the young.[5] It is their prevailing faith – and their sound practical logic – that allows Cree people to live with the unresolved contradictions surrounding the foods and other products that are being imported to and consumed by their community.

Another direct threat to *miyupimaatisiiun* is the lessons of 'proper' nutrition being taught to Cree adults at the medical clinic. The discussion of 'proper' nutrition across cultural fences brings to the fore contentious issues of power and authority. To suggest that there is a better way to eat is to imply that what the Cree have been doing for centuries is wrong and that what the clinic staff are teaching is right. This leads to confusion and uncertainty. For example, some women wanted to know how eating fat can be bad for people. For the Cree, fat is such a highly valued foodstuff that to consider it harmful verges on outrageous. In much the same way, to have excess fat on one's body is, for the Cree, a sign of well-being, not a harbinger of future ailments. This conflict is illustrated by a study which found that 100 per cent of the clinic staff felt that obesity was a significant health problem for the James Bay Cree, while only 29 per cent of the community health representatives agreed with this position (Lavallée, 1987).

Could it be, some asked, that weakened health has more to do with the *quantity* of whiteman's food now being eaten? Eating whiteman's food to excess was likened to consuming alcohol to excess: both the foods and the alcohol are relatively new to the Cree; both were introduced by whiteman; and both lead to disease when taken in large quantities. As one individual remarked, the risks associated with both are thus neither fully known nor fully understood.

Examples of whiteman's encroachment are found in many other realms of daily life in Whapmagoostui. The new housing facilities are often viewed with disdain. Despite the conveniences associated with them, some individuals consider the new dwellings completely unsatisfactory:

I feel much better when I live on the land and in a dwelling one lives in, than I feel when I am living inside a house. Even though I know that the house gives me comfort and shelter I feel much healthier and I have a sense of well being when I am on the land and living in an Indian dwelling. When I am outside, I feel a sense of well being and I feel that being out there helps me a great deal in feeling well and fine.

As an abstraction, *waamistikushiiu* carries a strong negative charge. Whiteman is viewed as having imposed a host of restrictive practices on the lives of the Cree, and as having overwhelmed traditional forms of education and spirituality. The seemingly endless battles against hydro-electric projects only serve to confirm this long-established fact among the people of Whapmagoostui.

Cree Cultural Identity

It is important to remember that though the Eastern Cree have long been connected by blood and marital ties, the Cree *nation* is a modern political construct. It has emerged over the past two decades to fill the need for a stable, cohesive unit that can react to issues relating to the control and development of the natural resources of the Cree lands in northern Quebec. Through the Grand Council of the Crees of Quebec (GCCQ), the nine Eastern James Bay Cree communities speak with a unified political voice and present a unified national identity in their economic, political, and 'cultural' battles with Quebec. In a bit of ironic play, I borrow from Handler's work on Quebec nationalism to explain the enduring 'culture war' between the Eastern Cree and the Quebec government: 'Despite bitter disagreements, the disputants in contemporary "culture wars" share an understanding of what cultural property is; that is, all disputants – current, would-be, and former imperialists, as well as oppressed minorities, ex-colonies, and aspiring new nations – have agreed to a world view in which culture has come to be represented as and by "things"' (1988: 157–8). For the Cree (as for the Quebec nationalists) those 'things' include all the stuff of historical and contemporary life: beliefs, language systems, ways of living in the world, and material objects. They are all the things that people point to first when they are justifying and validating a particular identity in the world (cf. Thomas, 1992; Kapferer, 1988). For the Whapmagoostui people, cultural property defines the Cree and distinguishes them from non-Cree; it also establishes what Cree identity means in the face of expansive northern development.[6] In Whapmagoostui, I am interested in how those 'things' of culture are negotiated, represented, incorporated, and enacted in everyday life – more specifically, in how they are connected to a Cree sense of 'being alive well.' Let me offer two specific examples.

In many Whapmagoostui households the radio is tuned to the local Cree station and is left on for a good part of the day. The station, which broadcasts entirely in the Cree language, is an important communication medium. For one hour in the morning and again in the late afternoon, news and information is fed live from CBC Northern Services (based in Montreal) to all the Eastern Cree communities. The rest of the day and evening, the radio transmits local programs – mostly country and western or rock music interspersed with local news and public service announcements. The radio is also used as a message relay centre. Finally, it runs twice-weekly bingo games, a vital source of revenue for this small enterprise.

The radio is a powerful medium for sustaining in the public consciousness those issues which reflect problems as stemming from whiteman's interference. For example, regular health and safety announcements are made on the radio. The issues touched on by these announcements range from water safety to the dangers of consuming certain species of fish or the organ meats of large game because of possible mercury or cadmium contamination. These latter warnings serve a direct purpose by advising people about potential hazards; at the same time, they support the conviction that the Cree face impediments arising from *waamistikushiiu*'s mismanagement of natural resources (cf. R. Scott, 1997; Archibald and Kosatsky, 1991). Thus in everyday life the distinction is sustained between *waamistikushiiu* and the Cree people.

My second example draws from the practices at Whapmagoostui's local school. At Badabin Eeyou elementary and high school,

Cree culture and Cree language are part of the basic curriculum. While children are raised with Cree as their first language, Cree language classes offer the only opportunity for them to learn the syllabarium. As well, there are Cree 'culture' classes, divided by gender, which offer boys and girls some of the basic skills they need to produce valued 'traditional' objects. Boys are taught how to construct such things as wooden sleds and snow shovels; girls learn how to sew and decorate items such as gun sacks and ammunition bags (to be used by the men), and how to cook bannock and other *iyimiichim* (Cree foods). Boys' culture classes are held in a room that looks like a wood-working shop; girls' classes are held in the 'Girl's Cree Culture' room, a home economics setting. The classes, which are taught entirely in the Cree language by local men and women, reinforce the notion that Cree culture is based mainly on material goods such as snowshoes, sleds, and snow shovels; they also sustain the strict gender categories of women's and men's work in traditional Cree society. In school, then, Cree culture and tradition are presented as something tangible. Yet the contemporary enactments of 'tradition' in a structured school setting reinforce a particular, and particularly artificial, sense of what it means to 'be Cree.'

Fortunately, classroom activities constitute only part of the Cree people's efforts to reinforce what it means to 'be Cree.' For good example, children are exposed to bush living and hunting from an early age. Also, more recently they are participating in annual summer gatherings and Cree culture camps, which are specifically geared to (re)invigorating Cree ways (Adelson, 1997). These present-day 'traditional' activities are enlivened with images of the past drawn from various stories, which are recounted to the children. In much the same way as I was told a variety of stories and cautionary tales in the interview context, adults, children, and grandchildren are regularly regaled with stories of mythic creatures, legendary heroes, and great successes and tragedies of the past. Sometimes the stories are told at bedtime, and sometimes at general meetings or other public events, and sometimes simply while sitting and having a cup of tea in the warmth of a tent or tipi. These stories and tales lend present-day traditional activities a symbolic potency and link them strongly to the past (C. Scott, 1991, pers. comm.; Connerton, 1989). As I explained in the previous chapter, these stories provide the images that are evoked in descriptions of *miyupimaatisiiun*. The resulting sense of identity is integral to – and inseparable from – one's sense of 'being alive well.'

The Limits of *Miyupimaatisiiun* and the Assertion of Political Well-Being

In their discussions of the ideals of Cree well-being, men and women offered a vision of a world in which whiteman's interference was minimal. That world is constituted primarily in the past, during a time when there were fewer outside influences on the adults and children. Life may have been harder during that time, and fewer may have survived, but the hardships endured were within the scope of those who lived off the land the year round. Misfortunes were primarily the result of fluctuations in the availability of animals, or of the arduous lifestyle of those who lived in the bush.

The ideals of *miyupimaatisiiun* are linked to what the Cree consider a healthy lifestyle: living in the bush and partaking in all that bush life offers. Today, bush camp, goose hunting, and bush-related activities are more than 'what Cree do'; they reaffirm the distinction between Cree and whiteman. Recall the bitterness in Elizabeth's voice as she called into the sky, decrying the scouting activities of the Hydro-Quebec surveyors. The helicopter was not just scaring away the geese; it was also directly threatening a social space that is not meant to include the people or activities associated with a modern southern economy.

Without a doubt, the bush is a special place – both a space and a time for people to live outside the structures and constraints of the village. Realistically, however, most of the Whapmagoostui Cree can only live in the bush at certain times of the year, as most work and live in the village. The exception is the biannual goose hunts, when Whapmagoostui is emptied as families head out to their respective hunting camps. Also, many families have winter and summer weekend camping sites within an hour's travel of the village. And, of course, many men and young boys enjoy heading out in search of caribou, or smaller game such as rabbits and ptarmigan. Most members of the community are not opting to return to full-time bush living. While some people still aspire to this ideal, many feel that some combination of village and camp life is a more realistic proposition.

Village life is associated with such things as structured schooling for the children, and with all the harm and disruption arising from alcohol consumption, and is viewed as negative and upsetting, and as offering none of the social peace that is associated with bush living. By and large, the community views the changes arising from village life as damaging, or at the very least as not conducive to 'being alive well.' Inexplicable ills have come to be associated with town life,[7] and so have problems among youth such as drug and alcohol abuse and vandalism. The latter problems are perceived by the elders as particularly difficult, and some admit they are at a loss to solve them.

There is one thing I am worried about that could put the Iyiyuu of today in a bad situation. The thing I am leery of is what has happened to other native communities when the waamistikushiiu comes into or comes within the surrounding area of the native community. Always without exception, the waamistikushiiu brings certain habits and one example is drinking. I can not say that I reject everything that the waamistikushiiu brings but what it does to the Iyiyuu. That is what makes me fear that these kinds of things will make trouble or make the Iyiyuu go the wrong way.

When I am outside[in the bush], I feel a sense of well being and I feel that being out there helps me a great deal in feeling well and fine. It also helps me to feel fine when I am doing the work that one does when one is in camp. The other thing that I have found out is that it helps one to be on the land because it is always clean and pure out on the land. Wherever the person is, it is always clean and pure. That is what helps the person for his well-being.

The announcement of a hydro-electric project only heightened concerns already held by the people about the potential threat to their land base. To not 'be alive well' is not necessarily to be sick, but rather to be in circumstances other than those envisioned as ideal. If, as I have suggested, Cree foods, land, hunting traditions, and lifestyles are all integral to *miyupimaatisiiun*, then the exploitation of indigenous lands and people would logically be the most profoundly felt impediments to Cree well-being. This was especially true in 1990, when people were stepping up their fight against the Great Whale hydro-electric project. Heightened threats to the land intensified the struggle to affirm control of that land and magnified its value and importance in the lives of the people. While the links between Cree lives and *miyupimaatisiiun* were already obvious in the interviews I conducted months before the project was announced, the sentiments arising from those links only deepened as my fieldwork progressed in the wake of the government's announcement.

If one objective of the social sciences is to 'look ... through the so-called normal arenas of political power and control' (Bourdieu, 1977: 189; Comaroff, 1985a), then this local examination of the meanings of 'health' takes on particular added value. In *miyupimaatisiiun* we see a distinctive form of agency, in the sense that through 'being alive well' people are articulating dissent through cultural assertion. Health and identity are linked as part and parcel of the ongoing struggle for voice and endurance in a world that has, over the years, muted and disenfranchised native people's existence.

'Being alive well' is a means by which adult Cree can articulate their distinct status in opposition to the persistent encroachment of whiteman upon themselves and their land. More specifically, 'being alive well' incorporates references to the past, and concentrates issues of identity around a particular set of cultural beliefs and practices in such a way that this assertion of health speaks to ideals that can only be enacted through that which is immediately understood as 'being Cree.' This is why we must understand, for example, that eating Cree food is not just an internally consistent cultural practice, nor is it merely something that symbolically or physiologically affects the nature of Cree individuals. Rather, eating Cree food imbues everyday practice with political process.

If there had been no 'New World' discoverers, no fur traders, no missionaries, no government assistance, and no provincial resource management projects, would the Cree people be describing *miyupimaatisiiun* in the same way today? Have the Cree always harked back to the 'good old days' – days when the water was cleaner and the animals were better to eat? Will the Cree children of today reminisce about the 1990s as the 'good old days' when they are their grandparents' age? For obvious reasons, these questions are impossible to answer. But perhaps one can speculate that with each perceived threat and each metre of encroachment, the Cree people's sense of identity grows more and more coherent, and in such a way that traditional notions of culture, however they are understood and recreated, become an increasingly important avenue of self-perception and, it follows, self-presentation. Thus the question is no longer, 'How can health be related to land and identity?' Instead, the question is, 'How can it not?'

Chapter 5

Summary and Postscript

I began this treatise on the bio-politics of health with a quote from Joseph Masty Sr. 'How,' he asked during one of our interviews, 'can we be healthy if the land is not?' That question could just as easily have moved me into the realm of political ecology or environmental health. Instead, I focused on what health means to the Whapmagoostui Cree in the context of their symbolic, economic, political, and historic relations with the land and, more generally, with the State. There is no doubt in my mind, however, that the question is more complex than this, even as I limit my ruminations to its anthropological implications.

Early on, and owing in a large part to Mr Masty's question, I rejected an implicit biomedical interpretation of health. At the same time, I did not limit my analysis of *miyupimaatisiiun* to its symbolic or representational forms. Along with all of its rich cultural meanings, this Cree concept of 'health' is also a component in larger strategies of identity and of dissent. Of course, I continue to underscore the fundamental difference between health and *miyupimaatisiiun* when health is used simply to describe biological phenomena or to represent a series of population norms. Yet just as health can be explored as an avenue of resistance (Crawford, 1985; Das, 1990; Lupton, 1995), so too can *miyupimaatisiiun*. Thus, I have situated these representations of *miyupimaatisiiun* within a particular form of political discourse suggested by the Cree themselves – one in which the politics of land are mediated through the landscape of the body.

Given that the body 'is the point at which individual experience and collective ideologies intersect' (Das, 1990: 43; Lindenbaum and Lock, 1993; Lock and Scheper-Hughes, 1990), it is not surprising that struggles are played out through interpretations of health. As I have shown, strategies of health can be strategies of dissent, or at the very least the means by which a person, through his or her body, can become involved in the negotiations of power between the State, the disenfranchised group, and the individual. For the Whapmagoostui people, strategies of health – *miyupimaatisiiun* – connect individual bodies to that larger political process; in this way links are formed between health, cultural assertion, and dissent within both individual bodies and the body politic.

Postscript

Since I completed my initial study, there has been a fusion of health and politics arising from an unanticipated confluence of anthropological data and Cree practical logic. Not too long after I completed the research and analysis, I disseminated the information back to the Cree people. I distributed copies of the research results to the Whapmagoostui Band Council, the Cree Regional Board of Health and Social Services, and the Grand Council of the Cree of Quebec, as well as to some individual members of the Whapmagoostui community. I also did a regional radio interview. To be sure, the term and concept *miyupimaatisiiun* was quite familiar to the Cree themselves. My intention was to present it to the people in a slightly differently light, refracted through the lens of critical-interpretive medical anthropology. As I soon discovered, a concept emerged that resonated with potential. What I want to point to here, in these final pages, is not so much that my work is being used, but the way in which the concept of *miyupimaatisiiun* has come to signify a position of 'self' (irrespective of *how* it is being used). Such marks of difference, as Bhabha says, 'inscribe a "history" of the people [and] become the gathering points of political solidarity' (1990: 306).

The first use of my research on *miyupimaatisiiun* was in an introductory guide for medical personnel arriving in the Cree region for the first time. *The James Bay Experience: A Guide for Health Professionals Working among the Cree of Northern Quebec* orientates new health care workers to the communities and the available facilities; it also offers a brief organizational history of the Cree Regional Board of Health and Social Services (CRBHSS) and a short account of the Cree people themselves, including their sense of 'health.' The concept of 'being alive well' is addressed only briefly in that guide; however, I have since learned that the term *miyupimaatisiiun* has been incorporated into the basic vocabulary to orient new doctors, dentists, and other health personnel. A woman at the health board told me that the term is important 'for the medical people to understand, and it has helped to verbalize a concept ... It has become part of the language of health education at the Cree Board because *it fits*. It's incorporated, for example, into teaching diabetes instructions ... It's quoted in a number of documents when they want to discuss a more holistic approach to health.'

In 1994 the research and education arm of the CRBHSS, the Module du Nord, produced a radio programmers' guide, *Miyupimaatisiiun: Promoting Health and Well-Being on Cree Radio*. This guide was compiled as an aid for local community programmers interested in researching and broadcasting radio programs on health issues. It begins with a definition of health (*miyupimaatisiiun*) that draws specifically from passages of my work. This concept of health sets the tone of the overall project, which according to the authors is intended to promote a holistic approach to health in the Cree region. The authors of this programming guide explain that *miyupimaatisiiun* embraces a number of perspectives. It would be wholly appropriate, they add, to discuss a range of health-related issues, be they of community-based or scientifically-based origins (Roth, Valverde, and Robinson, 1994).

A final example: the CRBHSS recently renewed its lobbying efforts to establish a public health department for the Cree region that would be administered directly by the board. As it stands now, the Module du Nord is based in Montreal and is linked to the public health arm of Montreal General Hospital.

For a long time, the CRBHSS has wanted to sever those connections and create an autonomous research and health promotion unit. The negotiations have been labyrinthine, and thankfully they are not relevant to the point I wish to make here. What *is* relevant however is that in the argument the board is making for a local northern health module, the distinctiveness of Cree 'health' is defined in English through the language of my work.

The Cree term *miyupimaatisiiun*, as 'unwrapped' by the anthropologist, has taken on new meanings and values that I never anticipated when I was conducting my initial research. Specifically, the often-quoted phrase, 'There is no Cree word that translates back into English as health,' has become a statement of political consequence. This phrase concretizes an abstraction – that is, it provides the language for sensitizing non-native health workers as well as for substantiating the political and economic autonomy of the CRBHSS. Originally, I defined Cree health in terms of an assertion of identity and dissent; yet the concept of health takes on new and added significance each time it is used to reaffirm distinctiveness and difference – in other words, each time it validates a particular (and particularly important) sense of what it means to be Cree. An alternative concept of health rooted in the community has expanded to become part of the language of the CRBHSS. In a way I could have never anticipated, health continues to be mediated by context, by history, and by culture; it is, in other words, deeply embedded within the language, practices, and processes of dissent.

Notes

1: 'If the land is not healthy then how can we be?'

1 In contrast to all other quotes, which retain the anonymity of the speaker, I am – with permission of his family – acknowledging Mr Joseph Masty, Sr as the person who so aptly summarized my entire project for me. Mr Masty, a respected elder in Whapmagoostui, died tragically a few short years ago. I offer his words in honour of his memory.

2 Whapmagoostui shares the same point of land as the Inuit village of Kuujjua-rapik. When referring to the general locale, I use the term Great Whale. Whapmagoostui is the term I use when referring specifically to the Cree community.

While some of what I talk about can be generalized to the Eastern James Bay Cree, I discuss specifically the Whapmagoostui Cree of Great Whale River, since that is where I conducted my research. As well, there is a confusion in the literature about the linguistic and cultural affiliation of the Great Whale Cree. They are alternatively referred to as Montagnais, or Naskapi, or Montagnais-Naskapi, or distinguished as entirely separate from either of these more eastern Algonquian groups. Affiliation with the Western Hudson Bay Cree was an accident of missionization when the assumption was that the populations on either side of James and Hudson bays were more closely related to each other than to groups to the east or west of the bays, respectively. Despite the closer affiliation to the Innu (Naskapi or Montagnais), religious and administrative links were determined through Moose Factory, and the term Cree was used to classify these peoples. I will follow the present-day usage of the terms Cree and Whapmagoostui Cree, along with the northern Cree nomenclature of *Iyiyuu* (sing.) and *Iyiyuu'ch* (plu.). *Iyiyuu* means 'person' and implies a native person and, in Whapmagoostui, specifically a Cree person.

3 Because they focus primarily on illness events, illness beliefs, and the clinical encounter, medical anthropologists have for a long time neglected the study of health (Kleinman, 1995). Yet in investigations limited to disease and illness, the focus of analysis has often been kept at the level of the illness experience and the clinical encounter; this perpetuates the mind/body dualism that is central to the biomedical model of disease and cure. The disease/illness distinction does not address or acknowledge the social relations inherent in illness or *health* processes – how, in other words, those experiences are shaped and distributed in society (A. Young, 1982). In much the same way that biomedicine focuses exclusively on individual disease phenomena, so too have medical anthropologists far too often restricted their studies to illness experiences and clinical processes.

4 See Adelson (1992) for a thorough review of health theories in the social sciences.

5 Kass points out that the word *health* is rooted etymologically in the Old English (*hal*) and Old High German (*heil*) words for *whole*; 'to be whole is to be healthy, and to be healthy is to be whole' (1981: 15). The word *health* has no root relationship to the words for disease, illness or sickness (1981: 15).

6 '"Healthiness",' laments Lupton, 'has replaced "Godliness" as a yardstick of accomplishment and proper living' (1995: 4). Conrad (1994) examined this link between morality and health and found that among American college youth the 'wellness revolution' has become a central trope in the playing out of a moral discourse. The body, in other words, has become a visible measure of moral worth; 'health is such a dominant value, [that] the body provides a forum for moral discourse and well-ness seeking becomes a vehicle for setting oneself among the righteous' (1994: 398; Litva and Eyles, 1994). This, of course, narrowly defines a particular way of understanding health – profoundly circumscribed by the awkwardly homogenous category of 'Western' and for the most part, middle class. It is a pervasive discourse, however, and certainly deserves attention as a distinct example of how health is constructed within and through the social order.

7 See Lupton (1995) for an excellent historical and sociological treatise on the relationship between public health discourses and the social, historical, and political settings out of which they emerge.

8 A new plan was recently announced by the Quebec provincial government and Hydro-Quebec. Rather than build new turbines and the necessary accompanying infrastructure so far north, the plan is to divert the Great Whale River south to a reservoir already in existence as part of the James Bay I project. The Whapmagoostui people held a referendum on 28 July 1997 and voted overwhelmingly to fight this new incarnation of the hydro-electric

project. It is not clear at this point if provincial Cree leaders will be as willing or as able to fight this project as they were the first time around.

9 As in any other study, there are limitations in the extent to which one can generalize from this analysis. As I detail later, the people with whom I spoke were primarily the elders and older adults from a small, northern Cree community. Their interpretations and discussions of *miyupimaatisiiun* may or may not resonate with the younger generations – or for that matter, with Cree people from other communities.

10 My new little daughter has already added another dimension to my work and social life in Whapmagoostui. As I write this, we have just returned from her first summer in Whapmagoostui. My role as mother was closely observed and quickly critiqued when it appeared that I had not properly protected my daughter from the frigid winds that blow off Hudson Bay.

11 Once established in the Cree community, I was perceived as one of 'them' by the predominantly French-speaking 'white' community. In this case, language was not the distinguishing factor, but that I associated exclusively with the Cree population.

2: The Whapmagoostui *Iyiuu'ch*

1 In January 1995 the Whapmagoostui Band census indicated a population of 604: 307 men and 297 women. There was a disproportionate split between young and old: 406 or 67 per cent were under 30 (188 of these were 10 or younger) and 198 (33 per cent) were over 30.

2 The airport is provincial property, expropriated by the government from Inuit category 1A land. There is a widely acknowledged need for radar facilities to assist landings, but more land is needed for this. Negotiations between the government and the Inuit have been stalled by the debates surrounding the hydro-electric projects. One of the 'carrots' offered to the native people was a new airport to be built a short distance away from the communities. Another carrot was a road to connect the community to the rest of Canada. Neither was mentioned again after the project was halted.

3 The Cree term that corresponds to the calendar month of August is *chiimaan piisim*, which translates as 'big boat month.' Back in the 1960s this was a month to look forward to, since the incoming ships needed men to help unload the cargo. Up and down the coast, men were hired to do this work, thus guaranteeing some summer income. More recently, barges and boats are bringing cars, trucks, and supplies for the residents of Great Whale.

4 Animistic spiritual beliefs ran counter to the early teachings of the missionaries. Consequently, many of the tales have been either lost or suppressed

because of the silence imposed on past generations by the authority of the early Christian leaders. Yet the (his)story-telling tradition – and indigenous spirituality – are very much alive in Whapmagoostui, and recently there has been a successful campaign to recall and record the legends and tales of the past.

5 The spirit guide, or *mistaapaau*, is a spirit intermediary with whom one communicates in, for example, a shaking tent ceremony. For a fuller explanation of the shaking tent ceremony and *mistaapaau*, refer to Chapter 3, note 14.

6 In Cree the word for person is the same word that distinguishes one Cree person from another. Thus, *Iyiyuu* (*Iyiyuu'ch*, pl.) indicates that one is referring to any person or, in particular, a Cree individual. The term *Iyiyuu* can also be used to distinguish between Cree and other indigenous groups, or between indigenous and nonindigenous people, or between a living person and other living creatures, such as animals.

7 Chisasibi, the second-largest of the Cree communities, is about 200 kilometres south of Whapmagoostui. The other coastal communities are Wemindji, Eastmain, and Waskaganish. The inland communities are, from north to south, Nemaska, Waswanipi, Mistissini (the largest of the Cree villages), and Oujé-Bougamou.

8 It should be noted that the period from early contact to the time of intense trade was marked by the introduction of catastrophic infectious diseases (e.g., measles, smallpox, influenza, scarlet fever, and tuberculosis) and by long periods of famine. It is believed that it was the Europeans who first carried these diseases into the trading regions, thereby infecting a population that lacked natural immunities (T.K. Young, 1988b, 1979). These 'virgin soil epidemics' had direct and indirect effects on the native populations. Added to the direct loss of a high number of adults in their prime years were the losses attributed to the reduction in the number of people responsible for food procurement, defence, and procreation (T.K. Young, 1988b; see also Jennings, 1976; Krech, 1978). When epidemics coincided with natural declines in animal populations, as occurred in the early 1900s, famine and disease were especially severe (Robinson, 1985).

9 In other cases 'the gatherings were shifted to the post locale to combine the practical, congenial and ideological goals of trade and social exchange' (Preston, 1975: 329).

10 The Hudson's Bay Company (HBC) men were the first European traders to come to the east coast of James Bay. Although they arrived in 1668, trade between the Cree and the HBC was not firmly instituted until the early 1700s. The first post on Hudson Bay was established at Richmond Gulf in the 1740s, with a smaller outpost at Little Whale River. This post lasted for ten years, after which time there were trading posts at either Fort George (estab-

lished in 1803) or the Little or Great Whale rivers (Morantz, 1983). For a complete review and analysis of trade relations with the Eastern James Bay Cree up to 1870, see Francis and Morantz (1983).

11 The Anglican missionaries followed the posting routes and went first to Little Whale and eventually to Great Whale River in the mid to late 1800s. The first permanent mission in this region was established in August 1879, when materials were shipped up to the Little Whale River for the construction of a church. The church was dismantled a few years later and moved by sled to the Great Whale River (Balikci, 1959). The church and mission activities brought a considerable number of coastal people to the region between the Great Whale River and Richmond Gulf (Francis and Morantz, 1983).

12 Many Cree now accept only the Christian teachings and have demoted indigenous spiritual practices, such as the shaking tent or sweat lodge ceremonies, to an archaic belief system. Others are reinvigorating their own religious practices, bringing Cree ceremonies out into the open for the first time in many, many decades. The changes in religious beliefs and practices are part of the contemporary changes occurring at Whapmagoostui, and properly belong in future writings.

13 Peck arrived in the eastern Hudson Bay region in 1876 and was soon followed and eventually replaced by Walton. From 1892 to 1924, Reverend W.G. Walton visited the Great Whale post regularly from Fort George (Petersen, 1974). In his absence there were Cree catechists trained to conduct the daily services.

14 Regular non-native visitors to Great Whale included the Mounted Police (twice-annual patrol), the HBC supply boat, the federal Indian agent, bush pilots, and the Field Medical Unit, which came by boat from Moose Factory about once a year. Less frequent visitors to Great Whale included naturalists, geologists, sportsmen, prospectors, and anthropologists (Honigmann, 1951, 1962; Walker, 1953).

15 For a comprehensive analysis of Cree systems of reciprocity, see C. Scott (1989). The idea that the post and the government were one and the same originated much earlier, about 1925, when the government provided some 'relief in kind' to the native population, to be distributed through the HBC. As Wills explains, 'learning that the Government provided the goods, the Indians now had a locus of origin established for the goods which originated in the south ... [Further,] if one sends furs south to receive goods, and if the Government sends goods north, then the furs must be received by the Government. And if a great deal of profit is made on the furs, then that profit goes to the Government' (1965: 57).

16 With the unique situation of so many Euro-Canadian residents appearing at one time at Great Whale, this was a period of intensive study of the inter-

ethnic relations and associations between communities. Graduate students (primarily), working under the tutelage of John Honigmann, conducted acculturation studies among the Cree and Inuit that focused mainly on the sudden influx of non-natives and their 'town' (Berger, 1974; Walker, 1953; Rogers, 1965; Wills, 1965). A pervasive racism runs like a thread through these studies. I was particularly struck by how hostile the non-native people were, especially to the Cree (Walker, 1953; Barger and Earl, 1971).

17 The barracks were soon turned into the region's first school, and later into a clinic, residences, and offices. A portion of the hangar eventually became Great Whale's first gymnasium. That first school was rudimentary at best, with classes held only in the summer months. Great Whale got its first day school in the 1960s, as more families came to live at the village site.

18 Barger (1977) notes that even after the DNA and the IAB were consolidated into the Department of Indian Affairs and Northern Development, the Inuit and the Cree were still administered separately.

19 For more comprehensive details of the dispute and of the negotiation process that resulted, see Feit (1985), Richardson (1977), and Salisbury (1986).

20 But as C. Scott (per. comm.) notes, to the extent that self-government is established as a right under the JBNQA, it has protection under Section 35 of the Constitution as a right established pursuant to a treaty or claims settlement, which is then an aboriginal right and hence 'inherent' in that sense, and not delegated.

21 The Cree Regional Authority was established in order to implement the policies of the GCCQ.

22 The establishment of the Cree School Board removed the Cree from the rivalry between the federal and provincial governments over educational jurisdiction in northern Quebec. The Cree School Board is funded provincially but holds full pedagogical control (Boulet and Gagnon, 1979).

23 Services were transferred to the control of the CRBHSS in 1978, and its offices were established in Chisasibi. Although it is modelled after and part of the Regional Council of Health and Social Services in Quebec, unlike other regional councils, the CRBHSS also manages a regional hospital centre (Chisasibi), a social service centre (Chisasibi), two reception and housing centres, and two local community service centres (Bobbish-Atkinson and Magonet, 1990). For a complete and concise summary of the complex organizational structure of the CRBHSS, see Bobbish-Atkinson and Magonet's *The James Bay Experience* (1990).

24 Category 2 lands are those upon which the Cree have exclusive hunting, fishing, and trapping rights, although the government retains the right to replace these lands with others if this is necessary in order to serve public

needs (e.g., mining). Category 3 lands are those on which the Cree hold no exclusive rights except to trap or hunt certain animals.

25 There is an increased emphasis among the Inuit on educating their children in French, so there is even less communication now between the younger generations of Cree and Inuit; the Cree speak Cree and English; the Inuit, Inuktitut and French.

26 The only time that Cree and Inuit participate jointly in activities is when they occasionally attend the other community's feasts or games. There have been only a few intermarriages; more recently a number of couples are sharing in the raising of their Cree/Inuit children without necessarily marrying.
Despite this limited daily interaction, there is a mutual respect shown when a death occurs in either community. From the time the death is announced, until after burial in a shared cemetery, flags are lowered everywhere, and all social events – from bingo to showers and weddings to community feasts – are postponed.

There is also an established reciprocity between the Cree and the Inuit in the preparation of the dead. Although the origin of this practice is unclear, Inuit women come to wash and prepare a deceased Cree individual, and Cree women do the same for the Inuit. One individual suggested that perhaps this practice originated in the days when it was mainly the older and incapacitated Cree and Inuit who were living at the post. With fewer people in either group, most would be in mourning for the deceased. This courtesy, possibly at the urging of the missionary, may have developed as a result.

27 Although the Inuit were in the majority until a few years ago, there are now more Cree than either Inuit or non-native inhabitants. This shift change is the direct result of a recent exodus of almost half the Inuit population from Great Whale to Umiujaq. Umiujaq, about 100 kilometres north of Great Whale, is a village that was petitioned for by Kuujjuarapik Inuit as part of the compensation package in the JBNQA. The construction and eventual move to this coastal village took place in the early 1980s.

28 The Cree never could and still cannot own real estate in Whapmagoostui, the Category 1A land according to the JBNQA. These lands have been set aside for the exclusive use of the Cree, but Quebec retains ownership (transferred from the Crown). Since property cannot be owned outright by individuals, homes are allocated and administered through the Cree Housing Corporation.

Recently a row of low-cost, low-maintenance homes was built in Whapmagoostui. These homes are very basic, with only modest facilities; they provide young or virtually full-time trapping families with affordable village living until more permanent houses can be built.

29 By accident of history the Inuit medical clinic was for many years on Cree land, and the Cree clinic 'up the hill' and thus on Inuit land. In 1995, a joint clinic was built between the two villages, but services within the centre are still duplicated.

30 This is a misnomer. The proposed 'second phase' of the project involves only Hudson Bay, not James Bay.

31 The Nottaway-Broadback-Rupert (NBR) project, a much larger undertaking, remains a real and constant if apparently latent concern for the Grand Council of the Crees of Quebec. The NBR project is a plan, studied since 1964, to divert the Nottaway and Rupert Rivers into the Broadback River. The catchment basins would spread over approximately 6500 km², and eight power stations would generate a peak power of between 8400 and 8700 megawatts (Gorrie, 1990; Hydro-Quebec 1990).

32 The Cree and Inuit united for a brief but significant period of time when they jointly fought against the hydro-electric project. That unity soon fell apart, however, when the Inuit government chose to negotiate a financial settlement with Hydro-Quebec and the provincial government, which provided them with what they would have received had the project actually gone ahead – though this did not include money.

3: *Miyupimaatisiiun*: 'Being Alive Well'

1 Part of the task of translation is to impart a sense of the original structure of the language in this modified format. If the excerpts seem awkward or unpolished it is because I have tried – as much as is possible both in translation and in print – to retain something of the original voice of the language, including especially the repetitions that are inherent to Cree story telling.

2 For the purpose of this study, older adults, or elders, are those born prior to 1940, while younger adults are those born during or after 1940. In total, I interviewed just under 20 per cent of the entire adult population born before 1960. I interviewed a total of twenty-nine individuals, each between one and six times. More men and women in the category of older adults (born prior to 1940) participated. Some individuals in these categories chose not to participate because of time conflicts, or lack of interest in the project, or because they were out of town during the interview periods. Potential participants' names were selected from the band list, and these people were contacted initially by telephone. The general purpose of the interview was described to them at that time. Prior to the start of the first interview, each participant read and signed the consent form, which was written both in English and in Cree syllabics. In keeping with recently estab-

lished practice, people who agreed to participate were financially compensated for their interview time. Interviews with unilingual Cree speakers were conducted entirely in Cree, with a translator and myself always present. Those who spoke English conversed in the language of their preference. We translated the interviews prior to subsequent visits so that I could follow up on particular items or events that were recounted in the previous interview. The interviews were supplemented by a series of less formal discussions with other members of the community, which were held throughout the duration of the field work period.

3 In the Cree language, all nouns, verbs, and qualifiers are categorized according to whether the noun is animate or inanimate. The root word *pimaatisiiu* implies an animate being, hence one that contains a spirit. Thus, animals, plants, rocks, and even tents are animate. Humans as well as animals, natural objects, spirit beings, legendary figures, and God can all be *pimaatisiiu* or alive (Feit 1983).

4 The younger adults focused to a greater extent on aspects of physical fitness and food. While many discussed these in relation to Cree ideals, descriptions of *miyupimaatisiiun* were at the same time couched within and compared to terms of reference drawn from their knowledge of biomedical norms. However, both younger and older adults felt a certain degree of frustration with the lessons learned through the clinic, public health programs, and popular media such as television.

   People of all ages discussed concepts relating to physiological health as well as a vast number of Cree remedies and therapeutics. This was for a number of reasons, I believe. First, the Cree pharmacopoeia is a tangible subject that people could easily discuss, and they were always willing to demonstrate their vast knowledge of remedies. As well, when there was a lull in the conversation, the translators would often resort to asking about traditional therapies. This wealth of information will be left to another report, except to note that it is indicative of a widely held concern for biological wellness.

5 I use a generic 'he' in most of these translations. In the Cree language there is no gender distinction for pronouns. The listener knows who one is speaking about by the use of a person's name or by the context of the discussion.

6 Moose are new to this region of northern Quebec. The migration patterns of the moose have shifted farther and farther north as the vast hydro reservoirs encroach on their more southerly routes.

7 For example, the word for the protective cloth sheaths that women make for men's rifles is the same as the word for condom. There is a continuation of this metaphor in relation to male sexuality and hunting (e.g., 'sperm' and 'gun powder' share the same word, and so do 'he ejaculates' and 'he shoots';

see Scott, 1989b). There are also many allusions to hunting in men's discussions of sexual intercourse (Tanner, 1979). Thus, when a ten-year-old boy in Whapmagoostui killed his first caribou, he was amiably teased by the elder to whom he presented a token of the kill, who said that the boy was now a man and ready to marry – that is, to have sexual relations (see also Tanner, 1979). There is no similar relationship between hunting and sexual maturity for women.

8 *Grandfather* can mean either one's parents' fathers or another male elder in the community. All of one's parents' siblings are considered one's grandparents, and all elders consider the children of the community their grandchildren.

9 Besides family feasts and gatherings, there are many events and festivities that are prepared and celebrated by the entire community (for a discussion of Cree feasts, see also Tanner, 1979, 1984). Community feasts are held on Christmas Day, Easter Sunday, and New Year's Eve. Also, community feasts are held after a communal walking-out ceremony, and after wedding ceremonies, and to celebrate specific events such as a visit from the bishop or high school graduation, and to commemorate a successful hunting season. The killing of a bear merits a bear feast, attended primarily by the elders of the community. Smaller family gatherings and feasts are held to celebrate the principal Christian holidays as well as young children's birthdays, major anniversaries, and bridal and baby showers (the latter attended primarily by women and their young children).

10 According to this elder, the ptarmigan beak symbolized that a walking-out feast was being held, since the ptarmigan is the first bird of significant size that a child will kill. See footnote 19, below, for an explanation of the walking out ceremony.

11 She is translated both as the Lady Spirit of the Caribou and as the Lady Spirit of the Wildlife. Either name indicates her status as the highest power in the spirit world of the animals.

12 *Minituu* means 'spirit' or 'power.' Bouchard and Mailhot translate the Montagnais term *mantusch*, analogous to *minitush*, as meaning 'maleficent power' (1972).

13 It should come as no surprise that many of the descriptions and explanations were proffered in the form of stories or parables. Ong (1982) explains that in a primarily oral culture, proverbs and stories are patterned for ready recall, since thought and memory systems are intertwined such that 'language is a mode of action and not simply a countersign of thought' (32).

14 For the Cree, the *mistaapaau* functions somewhat like an intermediary between the human and spiritual worlds. During a shaking-tent ceremony, one's *mistaapaau* is called on in order to relay messages between the two

worlds (see Preston, 1977; Feit, 1983). The shaking-tent ceremony was for a long time central to Cree hunting and religious ideology; its purpose was to communicate with the animal spirits, often to request assistance in locating those animals and hence, food (Feit, 1983; Preston, 1977; Tanner, 1979). With the recent surge in native spiritual practices in places like Whapma-goostui, there have been attempts to revive the shaking-tent ceremony, although not without controversy in the community.

15 It was suggested to me that perhaps he fainted or in some way lost consciousness (i.e., of the natural world).

16 In other versions of this story, each animal tells the man exactly which part of his body they will be.

17 Nursing women are also advised that they should not consume any beaver broth. Ultimately, I was told, the baby will be consuming that broth and then may replicate the habits of this nocturnal animal and lose his or her ability to sleep well during the night.

18 Current advice to the Cree Regional Authority is that the organ meats do not represent enough of a risk that current consumption practices need to be altered (Archibald and Kosatsky, 1991: 22). Also, there is some debate as to precisely how risky mercury contamination is, and what its effects are on the Eastern James Bay Cree (R. Scott, 1997).

19 See Tanner (1979) for a discussion of the walking-out ceremony, a rite of passage held around the time of a child's first birthday. The walking-out ceremony symbolizes a child's entry into the world of the Cree people; for many, it is the first time that the child is allowed out of doors without layers upon layers of warm clothing, and the first time he is allowed to touch the ground.

20 The 'moss bag' not only nestled the baby but also held the sphagnum moss that was used as diapering material.

21 I use the terms 'steam tent' and 'sweat lodge' interchangeably, since they translate to the same word in Cree. Today, the sweat lodge is associated with native spirituality and is used for a variety of medicinal and healing purposes. The elders who discussed the *mitutisaan* with me were referring specifically to a steam tent that could be used as a heat treatment. Of course, the medicinal application of heat could only be carried out by those who had the power and knowledge to heal. But this is still quite different from how the sweat lodge is used today.

A number of different heat treatments were described to me. Depending on the type of ailment, the healer would choose either a complete sweat lodge (*mitutisaan*) or a 'partial' sweat lodge over one area of the body. Alternatively, dry heat was applied to a part of the body with either a hot stone or a bag of heated sand. In the sweat lodge, steam heat was produced by pouring water over heated stones. A medicinal moss was added to enhance the steam treatment. The smooth, dark stones found underwater were described as the best type, since they produced more steam when moss was used with them. I was also told of a treatment that consisted of blowing steam directly into a person's mouth or onto the affected area of the body. (The steam tent was also used to cleanse the individual both physically and symbolically in preparation for hunting; see Tanner, 1979.)

22 Terms which indicate that one is lacking in physical strength are related to particular bush activities; they can also indicate gender distinctions between those activities. For example, when a man is thin and too weak to walk, one could say he is 'too weak to dig a hole in the ice.' When a woman is weak, one might refer to her as 'too weak to chop wood.'

23 It must be noted that stories are recounted partly as a means of celebrating the Cree people's ingenuity, resourcefulness, and determination (C. Scott, 1991, pers. comm.).

4: The Politics of *Miyupimaatisiiun*

1 While there is certainly enough evidence of exchanges that are clearly exploitative, Colin Scott does remind us there were also many that actually, or by necessity, fell within the realm of a recognized system of reciprocity: 'Contrasting [Cree] evaluations of the Whiteman relate to somewhat distinct functions for the reproduction of Cree society. On the one hand, positive evaluations sometimes amount to putting a necessary relationship in an optimistic light – viewing the Whiteman as irredeemably exploitative would only entail demoralization ... and would ignore altruistic features of Whiteman ideology of potential benefit to Crees' (1989a: 83).

2 The moniker for *pwaatich* used to tease the children is *pwaachikii* (or 'bogeyman,' as it was translated to me).

3 *Nituhkuiin* translates to 'medicine' in English but refers mainly to medicines available through the clinic, as opposed to Cree remedies (*nuuhchimiiunituhkuiin*, translates as 'bush medicine'). By and large, whiteman's diseases can only be cured by taking *nituhkuiin*, or 'whiteman's medicine.'

4 This devaluation of 'whiteman's food' is by no means specific to the northern Cree. Studies among the Eastern Cree (Berkes and Farkas, 1978), and among the Western Algonquian and Métis (Wein, Sabry, and Evers, 1989), indicate a preference by adults – and in the latter case by younger people as well – for bush food over store-bought foods. Qualitative analyses of other indigenous groups reveal the same partiality for bush food and provide relevant cross-cultural comparisons. While I do not presume any sort of universality of indigenous attitudes toward non-native foods, these examples do

provide interesting parallels to my findings. For example, Garro reports that for the Anishnabe of southern Manitoba, store-bought food is considered inferior to bush foods. Garro cites a medical case history of a woman complaining of 'weak blood,' which included signs of fatigue and weakness. The woman characterized her episode as a 'whiteman's sickness' directly related to the fact that she had been without wild food in the recent past (1990: 434). In another example, Borré describes how the North Baffin Island Inuit rely on seal meat and blood as the 'rejuvenator of human blood.' Without a regular diet of seal meat, a person can become physically, emotionally, and spiritually weakened (1991: 54; see also Meehan, 1982).

5 An adjunct to this dilemma is that some individuals are astonished that the grocery store's nutritional pamphlets and posters advise them to *not* purchase certain items. As one person summarized: 'Why have them for sale to begin with if they are bad for you?'

6 A recent plan by the Quebec government to create a permanent francophone community in the heart of Cree country speaks directly to this issue. The Quebec government would like to settle 2,000 Hydro-Quebec workers in the North to boost the region's economic development. A GCCQ spokesman has branded this 'ethnic occupation' fuelled by separatist scheming (Aubry, 1997: A1).

7 During the initial weeks of my field research, a young man died tragically and incomprehensibly. This thirty-year-old suffered a fatal heart attack one evening. It was the first time people could recall a young person dying from something other than an accident, and it unnerved the entire community.

While no quantitative studies have been done to date, there seem to be more asthmatics in Whapmagoostui today than ever before. People commented to me about this, associating lung problems with what they feel to be inadequate ventilation in the village houses.

Bibliography

Adelson, Naomi. 1992. 'Being Alive Well': Indigenous Belief as Opposition among the Whapmagoostui Cree. PhD diss., McGill University.
- 1997. *Gathering Knowledge: Reflections on the Anthropology of Identity, Aboriginality, and the Annual Gatherings in Whapmagoostui, Quebec.* Aboriginal Government, Resources, Economy and Environment Discussion Paper Series (Series Editor: Regina Harrison), Discussion Paper No. 1.
Alexander, Jeffrey C. 1990. Analytic Debates: Understanding the Relative Autonomy of Culture. In: J. Alexander and S. Seidman, eds., *Culture and Society: Contemporary Debates*, 1–30. Cambridge: Cambridge University Press.
Archibald, Chris P., and Tom Kostasky. 1991. Public Health Response to an Identified Environmental Toxin: Managing Risks to the James Bay Cree Related to Cadmium in Caribou and Moose. *Canadian Journal of Public Health* 82: 22–6.
Arctic Circular. 1949. The Nutrition and Health of the James Bay Indian, 2(4): 43–5.
Armstrong, David. 1983. *Political Anatomy of the Body: Medical Knowledge in Britain in the Twentieth Century.* New York: Cambridge University Press.
Aubry, Jack. 1997. Chevrette Wants Hydro Community in North. *The Gazette* (Montreal), 10 September, A1, A2.
Baer, Hans. 1986. Sociological Contributions to the Political Economy of Health: Lessons for Medical Anthropologists. *Medical Anthropology Quarterly* 17(5): 129–31.
Balikci, Asen. 1959. Tensions Sociales à GWR. *Annales de l'Association Canadien-Français pour l'Avancement des Sciences* 24: 128.
- 1961. Relations Inter-Ethniques à la Grande Rivière de la Baleine, Baie d'Hudson, 1957. In *Contributions to Anthropology*, 1959, 64–107. Ottawa: National Museum of Canada, Bulletin No. 173.

Barger, W.K. 1974. Adaptation to Modern Life in the Canadian North. PhD diss., University of North Carolina.

– 1977. Inuit and Cree Adaptation to Northern Colonialism. Manuscript of chapter in Ernest L. Shudsky, ed., *Contemporary Political Organization of the Native North Americans* (1980). Washington: University Press of America.

– 1981. Great Whale River, Quebec. In J. Helm, ed., *Handbook of North American Indians: Subarctic*, Volume 6: 673–82. Washington: Smithsonian Institution.

Barger, W.K., and D. Earl 1971. Differential Adaptation to Northern Town Life by Eskimos and Indians of Great Whale River. *Human Organization* 30(1): 25–30.

Berkes F., and C.S. Farkas. 1978. Eastern James Bay Cree Indians: Changing Patterns of Wild Food Use and Nutrition. *Ecology of Food and Nutrition* 7(3): 155–72.

Bhabha, Homi. 1990. DissemiNation: Time, Narrative, and the Margins of the Modern Nation. In H. Bhabha, ed., *Nation and Narration*, 291–322. London: Routledge.

Black, Mary. 1977. Ojibwa Power Belief System. In R.D. Fogelson and R.N. Adams, eds. *The Anthropology of Power*, 141–51. New York: Academic Press.

Black-Rogers, Mary. 1986. Varieties of 'Starving': Semantics and Survival in the Subarctic Fur Trade, 1750–1850. *Ethnohistory* 33: 353–83.

Bobbish-Atkinson, Helen, and Gordon Magonet. 1990. *The James Bay Experience.* Quebec: Government of Quebec.

Borré, Kristin. 1991. Seal Blood, Inuit Blood, and Diet: A Biocultural Model of Physiology and Identity. *Medical Anthropology Quarterly* NS5(1): 48–62.

Bouchard, Serge, and José Mailhot. 1972. Structure du Lexique: Les Animaux Indiens. *Recherches Amérindiennes au Québec* III(1–2): 39–67.

Boulet, Elisabeth, and Jo Ann Gagnon. 1979. *Poste de la Baleine after the James Bay and Northern Quebec Agreement.* Ottawa: Environment Canada (James Bay and Northern Quebec Office).

Bourdieu, Pierre. 1977. *Outline of a Theory of Practice.* Trans. Richard Nice. Cambridge: Cambridge University Press.

Canguilhem, Georges. 1989 [1966]. *The Normal and the Pathological.* Trans. Carolyn R. Fawcett. New York: Zone Books.

Comaroff, Jean. 1985a. *Body of Power, Spirit of Resistance: The Culture and History of a South African People.* Chicago: University of Chicago Press.

– 1985b. Bodily Reform as Historical Practice: The Semantics of Resistance in Modern South Africa. *International Journal of Psychology* 20: 541–67.

Communiqué de Presse. 1990. Un Coalition sans Précédent pour Exiger une Commission Spéciale Itinerante et Indépendente sur l'Avenir Energique du Québec. 15 February.

Connerton, Paul. 1989. *How Societies Remember.* Cambridge: Cambridge University Press.

Conrad, Peter. 1994. Wellness as Virtue: Morality and the Pursuit of Health. *Culture, Medicine and Psychiatry* 18: 385–401.

Copas, Matthew. 1989. Cree Reject Power Plans. *Montreal Daily News*, 17 March, 8.

Crawford, Robert. 1980. Healthism and the Medicalization of Everyday Life. *International Journal of Health Services* 10(3): 365–88.

– 1985. A Cultural Account of 'Health': Control, Release, and the Social Body. In J. McKinlay, ed., *Issues in the Political Economy of Health Care*, 60–101. London: Tavistock.

– 1994. The Boundaries of the Self and the Unhealthy Other: Reflections on Health, Culture and AIDS. *Social Science and Medicine* 38(10): 1347–65.

Cree-Naskapi Commission. 1986. 1986 Report of the Cree-Naskapi Commission (Commissioner's 1st Biennial Report). Ottawa: Cree-Naskapi Commission.

Cree School Board. 1987. *Cree Lexicon: Eastern James Bay Dialects.* Mistissini: Cree School Board.

Das, Veena. 1990. What Do We Mean by Health? In John Caldwell et al., eds., *What We Know about Health Transition: The Cultural, Social and Behavioural Determinants of Health: Proceedings of an International Workshop* 1: 27–46. Canberra: Health Transition Centre, Australian National University.

Dick, Robbie. 1991. Personal Communication.

Douglas, Mary. 1966. *Purity and Danger: An Analysis of Concepts of Pollution and Taboo.* London: Routledge and Kegan Paul.

Driben, Paul. 1988. *The Generation of Power and Fear: The Little Jackfish River Hydroelectric Project and the Whitesand Indian Band.* Toronto: Ontario Hydro (A Supplement to Ontario Hydro's Little Jackfish Hydroelectric Project Environmental Assessment).

Dunn, Frederick. 1968. Health and Disease in Hunter-Gatherers: Epidemiological Factors. In R.E. Lee and I. DeVore, eds., *Man the Hunter,* 221–8. Chicago: Aldine.

Feit, Harvey. 1983. The Power to 'See' and the Power to Hunt: The Shaking Tent Ceremony in Relation to Experience, Explanation, Action and Interpretation in the Waswanipi Hunters' World. MS.

– 1985. Legitimation and Autonomy in James Bay Cree Responses to Hydro-Electric Development. In Noel Dyck, ed., *Indigenous Peoples and the Nation State: Fourth World Politics in Canada, Australia and Norway,* 27–66. St John's: Institute of Social and Economic Research of Memorial University.

– 1986. Hunting and the Quest for Power: The James Bay Cree and Whitemen in the Twentieth Century. In R.B. Morrison and C.R. Williams, eds., *Native Peoples: The Canadian Experience,* 171–207. Toronto: McClelland & Stewart.

– 1991. Gifts of the Land: Hunting Territories, Guaranteed Incomes and the Construction of Social Relations in James Bay Cree Society. In N. Peterson and T. Matsuyama, eds., *Senri Ethnological Studies 30*, 207–23. Osaka: National Museum of Ethnology.

Flannery, Regina. 1962. Infancy and Childhood among the Indians of the East Coast of James Bay. *Anthropos* 57: 475–82.

Foucault, Michel. 1975. *The Birth of the Clinic: An Archaeology of Medical Perception*. New York: Vintage Books.

– 1980. *Power/Knowledge: Selected Interviews and Other Writings 1972–1977*. Ed. Colin Gordon. New York: Pantheon.

– 1989. Introduction. In *The Normal and the Pathological*, by Georges Canguilhem. New York: Zone Books.

Francis, Daniel, and Toby Morantz. 1983. *Partners in Fur: A History of the Fur Trade in Eastern James Bay, 1600–1870*. Montreal: McGill-Queen's University Press.

Frenk, Julio, José L. Bobadilla, Claudio Stern, et al. 1991. Elements for a Theory of the Health Transition. *Health Transition Review* 1(1): 21–38.

Garro, Linda. 1990. Continuity and Change: The Interpretation of Illness in an *Anishinaabe* (Ojibway) Community. *Culture, Medicine and Psychiatry* 14: 417–54.

Gazette (Montreal). 1991. Quebec to Appeal James Bay Ruling. 16 March, A5.

Gorrie, Peter. 1990. The James Bay Power Project. *Canadian Geographic*, Feb. March, 21–31.

Grand Council of the Cree of Quebec (GCCQ). 1990. 1989/1990 Annual Report of the Grand Council of the Cree of Quebec and the Cree Regional Authority. Nemaska: GCCQ.

Hamilton, Graeme. 1991. 'Cree Celebrate First Victory but Know Battle Isn't Over.' *The Gazette* (Montreal), 29 June, B4.

Handler, Richard. 1988. *Nationalism and the Politics of Culture in Quebec*. Madison: University of Wisconsin Press.

Honigmann, John J. 1951. An Episode in the Administration of the Great Whale River Eskimo. *Human Organization* (Summer): 5–14.

– 1962. Social Networks in Great Whale River: Notes on an Eskimo, Montagnais-Naskapi and Euro-Canadian Community (Bulletin no. 178). Ottawa: National Museum of Man.

Hydro-Quebec. 1990. *NBR Complex 1*. Montréal: Hydro-Québec.

Janzen, John M. 1981. The Need for a Taxonomy of Health in the Study of African Therapeutics. *Social Science and Medicine* 15B: 185–94.

Jennings, Francis. 1976. *The Invasion of America: Indians, Colonialism, and the Cant of Conquest*. New York: W.W. Norton.

Johnson, William D. 1962. *An Exploratory Study of Ethnic Relations at Great Whale*

River (NCRC 62–7). Department of Northern Affairs and National Resources. Ottawa.

Kapferer, Bruce. 1988. *Legends of People, Myths of State: Violence, Intolerance and Political Culture in Sri Lanka and Australia.* Washington: Smithsonian Institution Press.

– 1989. Nationalist Ideology and a Comparative Anthropology. *Ethnos* 54(3/4): 161–99.

Kass, Leon R. 1981. Regarding the End of Medicine and the Pursuit of Health. In: A.L. Caplan, H.T. Engelhardt, Jr., and J.J. McCartney, eds., *Concepts of Health and Disease: Interdisciplinary Perspectives*, 3–30. (Reprinted from: *The Public Interest* 40: 11–42.) Reading: Addison-Wesley.

Kelman, Sander. 1980. Social Organization and the Meaning of Health. *The Journal of Medicine and Philosophy* 5(2): 133–43.

Kistabish, Richard. 1982. La Santé Chez les Algonquins. *Recherches Amérindiennes au Québec* XII(1): 29–32.

Kleinman, Arthur. 1995. *Writing at the Margin: Discourse between Anthropology and Medicine.* Berkeley: University of California Press.

Krech, III, Shepard. 1978. Disease, Starvation, and Northern Athapaskan Social Organization. *American Ethnologist* 5: 710–32.

Lacasse, Fernande. 1982. La Conception de la Santé Chez les Indiens Montagnais. *Recherches Amérindiennes au Québec* XII(1): 25–8.

Lavallée, Claudette. 1987. Evaluation of the Community Health Representatives Program Serving the James Bay Cree. Report to the Community Health Department (DSC) of the Montreal General Hospital.

Leith, C.K., and A.T. Leith. 1912. *A Summer and Winter in Hudson Bay.* Madison: Cartwell Printing.

Lindenbaum, Shirley, and Margaret Lock, eds. 1993. *Knowledge, Power and Practice: The Anthropology of Medicine and Everyday Life.* Berkeley: University of California Press.

Litva, Andrea, and John Eyles. 1994. Health or Healthy: Why People Are Not Sick in a Southern Ontarian Town. *Social Science and Medicine* 39(8): 1083–91.

Lock, Margaret. 1993. *Encounters with Aging: Mythologies of Menopause in Japan and North America.* Berkeley: University of California Press.

Lock, Margaret, and Nancy Scheper-Hughes. 1990. A Critical-Interpretive Approach in Medical Anthropology: Rituals and Routines of Discipline and Dissent. In T.M. Johnson and C.F. Sargent, eds. *Medical Anthropology: A Handbook of Theory and Method*, 47–72. New York: Greenwood Press.

Lupton, Deborah. 1995. *The Imperative of Health: Public Health and the Regulated Body.* London: Sage.

Manning, Peter K., and Horatio Fabrega. 1973. The Experience of Self and

Body: Health and Illness in the Chiapas Highlands. In George Psathas, ed., *Phenomenological Sociology*, 251–301, New York: Wiley.

Marsh, G. 1988. *The Canadian Encyclopedia*, 2nd ed. s.v. 'Whaling' by Daniel Francis; 'Glaciation' by N.W. Rutter. Edmonton: Hurtig Publishing.

Masty, Emily. 1995. Women's Three Generation Life History Project in Whapmagoostui, Quebec. Official submission to the Royal Commission on Aboriginal Peoples, Ottawa, Canada.

– 1989. Personal communication.

Masty, Emily, and Susan Marshall. [nd]. Native Dreams: Stories from the People of Whapmagoostui. Ms.

McElroy, Ann. 1990. Biocultural Models in Studies of Human Health and Adaptation. *Medical Anthropology Quarterly* NS4(3): 243–65.

McElroy, Ann, and Patricia K. Townsend. 1985. *Medical Anthropology in Ecological Perspective*. Colorado: Westview.

McKnight, John L. 1986. Well-Being: The New Threshold to the Old Medicine. *Health Promotion* 1(1): 77–80.

Meehan, Betty. 1982. Ten Fish for One Man: Some Anbarra Attitudes towards Food and Health. In Janice Reid, ed. *Body, Land, and Spirit: Health and Healing in Aboriginal Society*, 96–120. St Lucia: University of Queensland Press.

Moore, P.E., H.D. Druse, F.F. Tiskall, and R.S.C. Corrigan. 1946. Medical Survey of Nutrition among the Northern Manitoba Indians. *Canadian Medical Association Journal* 54: 223.

Morantz, Toby. 1983. 'Not Annuall [*sic*] Visitors': The Drawing in to Trade of Algonquian Caribou Hunters. In William Cowan, ed. *Actes du Quatorzième Congrès des Algonquinistes*, 57–73. Ottawa: Carleton University Press.

– 1986. Historical Perspectives on Family Hunting Territories in Eastern James Bay. *Anthropologica* NS28(1/2): 65–91.

Navarro, Vincente. 1980. Work, Ideology and Science: The Case of Medicine. *International Journal of Health Services* 10(4): 523–50.

Ngubane, Harriet. 1977. *Body and Mind in Zulu Medicine: An Ethnography of Health and Disease in Nyuswa-Zulu Thought and Practice*. London: Academic Press.

Nichter, Mark. 1989. *Anthropology and International Health*. Dordrecht: Kluwer Academic.

Ong, Walter J. 1982. *Orality and Literacy: The Technologizing of the Word*. London: Methuen.

Ouellet, M.-B., and L. Sutherland. 1988. Evolution of Health Care System in the James Bay Area. *Arctic Medical Research* 47(Suppl. 1): 330–3.

Petersen, Olive M. 1974. *The Land of Moosoneek*. Canada: Diocese of Moosonee.

Preston, Richard. 1975. Eastern Cree Community in Relation to Fur Trade Post in the 1830's: The Background of the Posting Process. In William Cowan, ed.,

Papers of the Sixth Algonquian Conference, 1974, 324–35. Ottawa: National Museums of Canada (Mercury Series).

– 1977. Cree Narrative: Expressing the Personal Meaning of Events. Canadian Ethnological Paper no. 30. Ottawa: National Museum of Man, Mercury Series.

– 1981. East Main Cree. In J. Helm. ed., *Handbook of North American Indians: Subarctic*, 196–207. Washington: Smithsonian Institution.

Richardson, Boyce. 1977. *Strangers Devour the Land: The Cree Hunters of the James Bay Area versus Premier Bourassa and the James Bay Development Corporation*. Toronto: Macmillan.

Robinson, Elizabeth. 1985. Health of the James Bay Cree. Report to the Community Health Department (DSC) of the Montreal General Hospital.

Rogers, Patricia. 1965. Aspiration and Acculturation of Cree Women at Great Whale. M.A. thesis, University of North Carolina.

Roth, Lorna, Clara Valverde, and Elizabeth Robinson. 1994. *Miyupimaatisiiun: Promoting Health and Well-Being on Cree Radio*. Montreal: Module du Nord.

Salée, Daniel. 1995. Identities in Conflict: The Aboriginal Question and the Politics of Recognition in Quebec. *Ethnic and Racial Studies* 18(2): 277–314.

Salisbury, Richard F. 1986. *A Homeland for the Cree: Regional Development in James Bay: 1971–1981*. Montreal: McGill-Queen's University Press.

Saltonstall, Robin. 1993. Healthy Bodies, Social Bodies: Men's and Women's Concepts and Practices of Health in Everyday Life. *Social Science and Medicine* 36(1): 7–14.

Scott, Colin. 1983. The Semiotics of Material Life among the Wemindji Cree Hunters. PhD diss. McGill University.

– 1984. Cree Reciprocity with the Whiteman: Myth, History, and the Ideology of Relations with the State (MS).

– 1989a. Ideology of Reciprocity between the James Bay Cree and the Whiteman State. In P. Skalník, ed., *Outwitting the State*, 81–108. London: Transaction.

– 1989b. Knowledge Construction among Cree Hunters: Metaphors and Literal Understandings. *Journal de la Société des Américanistes* LXXV: 193–208.

– 1991. Personal communication.

Scott, Richard. 1997. *Becoming a Mercury Dealer: Moral Implications and the Construction of Objective Knowledge for the James Bay Cree*. Aboriginal Government, Resources, Economy and Environment Discussion Paper Series (series editor: Regina Harrison). Discussion Paper No. 3.

Shils, Edward. 1981. *Tradition*. Chicago: Chicago University Press.

Speck, Frank. 1915. Some Naskapi Myths from Little Whale River. *Journal of American Folklore* 28: 70–7.

Tanner, Adrian. 1979. *Bringing Home the Animals: Religious Ideology and the Mode of Production of the Mistassini Cree Hunters*. St John's: Memorial University of Newfoundland, Social and Economic Studies No. 23.

Thomas, Nicholas. 1992. The Inversion of Tradition. *American Ethnologist* 19(2): 233–54.

Tsing, Anna. 1993. *In the Realm of the Diamond Queen*. Princeton: Princeton University Press.

Turner, Bryan S. 1985. The Practices of Rationality: Michel Foucault, Medical History and Sociological Theory. In R. Fardon, ed., *Power and Knowledge: Anthropological and Sociological Approaches*, 193–212. Edinburgh: Edinburgh University Press.

Turner, Lucien M. 1894. Ethnology of the Ungava District, Hudson Bay Territory. *Annual Report Bureau of American Ethnology*: 167–350.

Turner Strong, Pauline, and Barrik Van Winkle. 1996. 'Indian Blood': Reflections on the Reckoning and Refiguring of Native North American Identity. *Cultural Anthropology* 11(4): 547–76.

Twomey, Arthur, C., and Nigel Herrick. 1941. *Needle to the North: The Story of an Expedition to Ungava and the Belcher Islands*. Boston: Houghton Mifflin.

Vivian, R.P., C. McMillan, P.E. Moore, et al. 1948. The Nutrition and Health of the James Bay Indian. *Canadian Medical Association Journal* 59: 505–18.

Waldram, James B., D. Ann Herring, and T. Kue Young. 1995. *Aboriginal Health in Canada: Historical, Cultural, and Epidemiological Perspectives*. Toronto: University of Toronto Press.

Walker, Willard B. 1953. Acculturation of the Great Whale River Cree. MA thesis, University of Arizona.

Wall, L. Lewis. 1988. *Hausa Medicine: Illness and Well-Being in a West African Culture*. Durham: Duke University Press.

Wein, Eleanor, Jean Sabry, and Frederick Evers. 1989. Food Health Beliefs and Preferences of Northern Native Canadians. *Ecology of Food and Nutrition* 23: 177–88.

Wills, Richard H., Jr. 1965. Perceptions and Attitudes of the Montagnais-Naskapi of Great Whale River Concerning the Western World. MA thesis, University of North Carolina at Chapel Hill.

Worsley, Peter. 1982. Non-Western Medical Systems. *Annual Review of Anthropology* 11: 315–48.

Young, Allan. 1980. The Discourse on Stress and the Reproduction of Conventional Knowledge. *Social Science and Medicine* 14B: 133–46.

– 1982. The Anthropologies of Illness and Sickness. *Annual Review of Anthropology* 11: 257–85.

Young, T. Kue. 1988a. *Health Care and Cultural Change*. Toronto: University of Toronto Press.

– 1988b. Are Subarctic Indians Undergoing the Epidemiologic Transition? *Social Science and Medicine* 26(6): 659–71.

Index

ANTHROPOLOGICAL HORIZONS

Editor: Michael Lambek, University of Toronto

This series, begun in 1991, focuses on theoretically ethnographic works addressing issues of mind and body, knowledge and power, equality and inequality, the individual and the collective. Interdisciplinary in its perspective, the series makes a unique contribution in several other academic disciplines: women's studies, history, philosophy, psychology, political science, and sociology.

Published to date: